American
Medical
Association

Guide to
Home Caregiving

Other books by the American Medical Association

American Medical Association
Complete Guide to Men's Health

American Medical Association
Guide to Talking to Your Doctor

American Medical Association
Family Medical Guide

American Medical Association
Complete Guide to Women's Health

American Medical Association
Complete Guide to Your Children's Health

American Medical Association
Family Health Cookbook

American Medical Association
Guide to Your Family's Symptoms

American Medical Association
Handbook of First Aid and Emergency Care

American Medical Association
Essential Guide to Asthma

American Medical Association
Essential Guide to Depression

American Medical Association
Essential Guide to Hypertension

American Medical Association
Essential Guide to Menopause

American
Medical
Association

Guide to
Home Caregiving

Angela Perry, MD
Medical Editor

JOHN WILEY & SONS, INC.
NewYork • Chichester • Weinheim • Brisbane • Singapore • Toronto

Published by John Wiley & Sons, Inc.
Published simultaneously in Canada

Design and production by Navta Associates, Inc.

This publication is designed to provide accurate and authoritative information in regard to the subject matter covered. It is sold with the understanding that the publisher is not engaged in rendering professional services. If professional advice or other expert assistance is required, the services of a competent professional person should be sought.

The recommendations and information in this book are appropriate in most cases; however, they are not a substitute for medical diagnosis. For specific information concerning a medical condition, the AMA suggests that you consult a physician. The names of organizations, products, or alternative therapies appearing in the book are given for informational purposes only. Their inclusion does not imply AMA endorsement, nor does the omission of any organization, product, or alternative therapy indicate AMA disapproval.

Library of Congress Cataloging-in-Publication Data:

The American Medical Association guide to home caregiving
    p. ; cm
  Includes index.
  ISBN 0-471-41409-3 (paper : alk. paper)
  1. Home health aides. 2. Caregivers. I. Title: Guide to home caregiving.
II. American Medical Association.
  [DNLM: 1. Home Nursing—methods. 2. Caregivers. 3. Home Care Services. WY 200 A512 2001]
RA645.3 .A4595 2001
362.1'4—dc21   2001024710

Printed in the United States of America

10 9 8 7 6 5 4 3 2 1

American
Medical
Association

Foreword

At one time or another, most families find themselves making decisions about providing care for a loved one at home. Many older people provide care for a spouse who is ill, and increasing numbers of adult children are caring for aging parents. The *American Medical Association Guide to Home Caregiving* provides hands-on, step-by-step practical advice for the home caregiver. The book addresses the general aspects of caregiving as well as the specific tasks required for caring for a person with a particular illness such as Alzheimer's disease.

If you are considering being a caregiver, you will probably want to know the extent of the commitment you are making, the amount of work it will involve, the tasks and skills you will need to learn, and the tasks that you should delegate to health-care professionals. The *American Medical Association Guide to Home Caregiving* helps you make this important decision and gives you the support and encouragement you may need. We believe that the more information you have about caregiving, the more effectively you will be able to provide the care—and the more enriching and gratifying the experience will be for both you and the person you are caring for.

The American Medical Association offers you this information as part of a continuing effort to provide you and your family with practical, up-to-date medical information. You can find useful health information by visiting the AMA Web site at http://www.ama-assn.org; if you are looking for a doctor or want to find out if a doctor is board certified, click on Doctor Finder, where you can search for information by medical specialty or by a doctor's name.

The American Medical Association wishes you and your family the best of health.

American Medical Association

The American Medical Association

Robert A. Musacchio

Senior Vice President, Business and Membership

Anthony J. Frankos

Vice President, Business Products

AMA Press

Mary Lou S. White	*Editorial Director*
Patricia Dragisic	*Senior Managing Editor*
Donna Kotulak	*Managing Editor*
Steven Michaels	*Senior Editor*
Janis Pinson Forgue	*Copy Editor*
Claudia Appeldorn	*Copy Editor*
Mary Ann Albanese	*Image Coordinator*
Dawn Goldammer	*Image Coordinator*
Reuben Rios	*Editorial Assistant*
Roger Banther	*Editorial Assistant*

Medical Editor

Angela Perry, MD

Writers

Gina Freed, RN, MSN

Karen Titus

Illustration

Rolin Graphics Inc.

Acknowledgments

Joanne Schwartzberg, MD	*Medical Reviewer*
Rosalie Guttman	*Reviewer*
Alzheimer's Association	

Contents

Introduction

At one time or another, most families will need to provide home care for a family member who is ill, aging, or disabled. Sometimes, health problems such as the flu are temporary and familiar. At other times a loved one's health problems, such as Alzheimer's disease or a terminal illness, may be extremely difficult to manage. Whenever possible, a person who is ill, disabled, or recovering from surgery or serious illness should be cared for in his or her own home. Familiar surroundings can have a positive effect on a person's sense of well-being, which can lead to a quicker, more complete recovery or, in cases in which recovery is not expected, a better quality of life.

Home healthcare is one of the fastest-growing segments of the healthcare industry in the United States. A large portion of this care is provided to older Americans—those 65 or older—whose numbers are expected to increase dramatically in the next few decades. Many younger people, too, may need some type of home healthcare, either for the long term or short term. For example, a person recovering from an injury or surgery may require home healthcare for a few weeks or months. People who have chronic diseases, or who are disabled or terminally ill usually require long-term or, in some cases, permanent care.

In the past, many conditions required long-term hospitalization, but this is neither practical nor affordable today. Healthcare providers and insurers, eager to cut the rising costs of care, have found that, in many cases, it is more practical and far less costly to shift the focus of care to the home. In addition, advances in technology and improvements in home caregiving techniques have made it easier to provide high-quality care away from a centralized healthcare facility. As a result, home caregiving has become a common practice throughout the United States.

While there are many benefits associated with home caregiving, it takes careful planning, support, and patience to make it a rewarding experience for everyone involved. Although being a home caregiver can have a major impact on your life, it is helpful to remember that you are not alone. Many others are facing the same challenges, and caregiving techniques and services are continually being developed and improved to help make your job easier and more effective.

If your loved one is seriously ill or has been ill or disabled for a long time, you probably have had many conversations with doctors, nurses, and other healthcare professionals. You may be feeling confused, overwhelmed, and frustrated by your inability to get answers to all your questions. You may be having problems dealing with Medicare, Medicaid, or a private insurance company, or find yourself filling out countless forms and trying to determine which costs are covered and which are not. And you are probably experiencing a great deal of stress as you struggle with strong emotions. The *American Medical Association Guide to Home Caregiving* gives you essential, hands-on information to help make your caregiving experience rewarding for both you and your loved one.

1

Preparing for Home Care

Before you begin caring for a loved one at home, it's a good idea to consult with the other members of the caregiving team—such as doctors, nurses, therapists, social workers, and family members—to identify and develop an effective strategy. This strategy is referred to as a care plan. Each family's situation is unique, and family members will need to work together to develop the best plan to deal with their unique situation. The plan should be flexible enough to meet the continually changing needs of the person who is being cared for. You may have to learn through trial and error what works best for you. Although it is not always possible to predict the exact course of an illness or how a person will recover, it is a good idea to discuss expectations and potential problems in advance with all members of the home healthcare team. This will help you to develop a support network and the best care plan possible. Consider the following when developing your care plan:

- How long the illness is expected to last
- How the person's condition might improve or worsen
- Whether it is possible for the person to fully recover from his or her condition or illness
- Whether rehabilitation therapies—such as physical, occupational, or speech therapy—will be needed to promote recovery and who will provide these services, if necessary
- The specific medical emergencies that might occur and how these emergencies should be handled
- Caregiving adjustments you will need to make, such as changes in a person's medication or need for therapy

Setting Priorities and Goals

The best time to begin planning the transition from hospital care to home caregiving is shortly after a person has been admitted to the hospital. This is a good opportunity for you to determine the needs of your loved one, create a care plan, identify potential caregivers, assign caregiving responsibilities, and address the needs of the caregiver. Typically, a hospital social worker, primary care nurse, or case manager will be available to guide you through this transition and help you plan strategies for successful home caregiving. This will allow you, once your loved one leaves the hospital, to concentrate on providing the best care possible for him or her.

You might find it helpful to create a log or journal about your care plan to keep track of new developments or changes in your loved one's needs. Consider the following questions when developing your care plan, tailoring your answers to your unique situation:

- What types of care will your loved one require and what is the best way to provide them?
- Will he or she require 24-hour care?

- If you need to monitor health indicators such as blood pressure or blood glucose level, or administer and adjust medications, who will train you to perform these tasks? And whom can you contact for advice and assistance?

- Who will be part of your caregiving team and what roles will they play? You may need the services of a variety of people, such as doctors, specialists, visiting nurses, therapists, and home health aides.

- What type of care is available, and from which agencies? Is the care effective and dependable, and what are the costs?

- Will you need any special equipment, such as that used to provide oxygen or intravenous feeding? Find out what equipment you need, who will train you to operate it, what type of maintenance it requires, and who will provide maintenance for it.

- Will physical changes have to be made to the person's home to enhance his or her mobility and safety? For example, you may need to have ramps, railings, or electric lift chairs installed on stairways. Grab bars and handrails help make it safer to use the toilet or bathtub.

- Will the person need specialized equipment to help him or her perform daily tasks? Various useful devices, such as a handheld "reacher" that can help a person grasp objects that are out of reach, are available from drugstores and medical supply companies.

- Will pets in the home create any special problems? Experts acknowledge that pets are often regarded as family members, but some pet-related routines and behaviors may need to be adjusted to prevent accidents. For example, you might install a child safety gate to keep a dog from getting in the way of a person who is learning to use a walker.

- What are the person's likely transportation needs? You may be able to use your own car or van or you may need to use a specially equipped van. Transportation services are available at reasonable cost in many communities; ask your doctor or nurse for recommendations or check your phone book.

In most families who are caring for a loved one, a spouse, parents, siblings, or children provide most of the routine care, with assistance from various healthcare professionals and under the supervision of a doctor. Do not worry if you have had no practical experience as a caregiver. Caregiving requires common sense and a caring approach that most people are able to provide, and any basic caregiving skills that you do not have already will be easy to learn. Caregivers rarely need special skills, but if you do, you can be trained to perform even difficult tasks effectively. People who have experienced firsthand the challenges and rewards of home caregiving emphasize self-education as the key to providing quality care. Learn as much as you can about your loved one's illness or condition:

- Attend discussions with physicians and other members of your loved one's healthcare team. Write down questions and take notes or tape-record sessions with care instructors. Learning how to handle a serious illness or injury requires taking in a lot of new information that you may not easily understand or remember. If you feel your questions are not being addressed in these meetings, schedule a separate meeting to resolve them.

- Consider consulting a private clinical social worker, gerontologist (aging specialist), or other appropriate care provider. These people are trained to navigate the complex healthcare delivery system. They can come into your home, evaluate your family's needs, and help you get the support you need, such as a physical therapist, a household helper, or even a hospital bed. They may also be able to help you make a decision about a nursing home in your community that meets your loved one's needs.

- Use the services offered by local and national support groups and organizations, community outreach programs at nearby hospitals and other healthcare facilities, and help hot lines. Consult your local public library, bookstores, and the Internet for additional information and resources.

The basic goal of caregiving is to keep your loved one as clean, comfortable, and content as possible. Keep in mind that when a person is seriously ill, even the smallest problems may be upsetting and can seem overwhelming. By keeping things running smoothly, you enable your loved one to rest and remain optimistic.

Planning and Arranging the Room

When planning your loved one's room, consider how ill he or she is and how long you are likely to be caring for him or her. Arrange the room to make it as comfortable and convenient as possible for both the person who is being cared for and his or her caregivers. Here are some helpful tips:

- In a two-story house, it is probably better for a person to stay on the first floor. This will help keep him or her from feeling isolated and will eliminate a lot of trips up and down the stairs for you. This arrangement will also help prevent potentially serious falls.

- Place a single bed in the room so that it is accessible from both sides; making the bed and moving the person in bed will be easier. If possible, place the bed near a window so the person can see outside and feel more connected to the rest of the world. If you need a hospital bed with side rails, you can rent one from a medical supply company.

- Use a bedside table to keep medications, water, tissues, a whistle or bell (to call for assistance), and any other important items within easy reach.

- If the person can get out of bed but cannot get to the bathroom easily, you will need a commode (a portable chair that contains a removable bedpan). You can rent or buy one from a drugstore or medical supply company or, in some communities, borrow one from a local health agency or volunteer organization. If the person is confined to bed, keep a bedpan (and a handheld urinal for a male) near the bed at all times.

- Be sure that the temperature in the room is comfortable and the air circulation is adequate. You may want to leave a window open slightly to bring in fresh air or use a small fan to keep the air moving, but be careful to keep the room free of drafts.

2

Basic Caregiving Skills

Once your loved one is at home, you will need to put the plans you have made into action. From now on, your daily routine will focus on meeting the needs of your loved one.

Giving Medications

As a caregiver, you will probably be responsible for giving medications to your loved one. This may be as simple as occasionally providing aspirin to reduce pain or fever, or as complex as coordinating a wide variety of drugs with eating and sleeping schedules. Learn all you can about your loved one's medications, starting with the names of the drugs. It can be helpful to use a divided container to hold the person's medications for each day of the week. If the person is taking several medications, it may be helpful to keep a list of their names and a written schedule of daily doses of each so that you can check off each dose as you give it. The schedule should also include any specific instructions. For example, some drugs need to be taken on an empty stomach and others within an hour or two of eating a meal. Some medications can be taken together, while others cannot.

Gather the necessary information and instructions about each prescribed medication from your doctor or pharmacist, and make sure that you understand everything. You may want to ask the doctor or pharmacist the following questions:

- When should the medication be taken (with meals, first thing in the morning, at bedtime, or two times a day, for example)?
- For how long should the medication be taken (will refills be necessary)?
- What are the possible side effects and what should you do about them?
- About which side effects should you notify the doctor?
- Does the medication interact with any other medications, either prescription or nonprescription, that the person is taking?
- Should the person avoid certain foods?
- Do any of the medications have any long-term effects?
- Does the medication have any warnings regarding children, older people, people with substance abuse problems, or others?
- Does the medication come in various forms? For example, if your loved one has problems swallowing pills, ask if the medication is available as a liquid. If you are giving liquid medication, always measure the dose carefully, using a special measuring spoon or cup, if provided. Never guess at the correct amount. And when pouring the medication, hold the bottle with the label facing up so that any overflow does not make the label illegible.

Remember that all medications must be taken exactly as prescribed by the doctor. Never stop giving medication to your loved one without the doctor's permission. If your loved one refuses to take a particular medication, try to find out why. It may simply be that the medication tastes bad. If this is the case, you may be able to mask the taste by crushing it if it's a pill and mixing it with a pleasant-tasting food such as pudding, yogurt, or applesauce. This is also a helpful solution if the person has trouble swallowing tablets or capsules. Ask your doctor or pharmacist for recommendations.

It is also possible that your loved one may refuse to take his or her medication for emotional reasons. For example, he or she may be feeling depressed about his or her condition, or may be looking for a way to exert more control. Calmly discussing the situation with your loved one may help you identify the problem and determine the best way to resolve it.

WARNING: Sometimes a medication can cause an allergic reaction, producing symptoms such as hives, itching, a rash, or wheezing, or side effects such as nausea or dizziness. If your loved one has any of these symptoms, call the doctor immediately to determine if you should stop giving the medication. The doctor may need to adjust the dosage or change medications.

Some substances, such as certain foods, prescription drugs, over-the-counter drugs, or alcohol, when taken with some medications can interfere with the drugs' effectiveness or cause undesirable (and sometimes dangerous) side effects or interactions. Some vitamin and mineral supplements can alter the effects of a medication. Be sure to ask your doctor or pharmacist about potential interactions and reactions with any medications your loved one is taking.

Providing a Healthy Diet

Healthy eating is essential for maintaining your loved one's health and well-being and is also a factor in successful recovery from an illness or injury. A person who is confined to bed usually looks forward to mealtime, because eating is a pleasurable experience, helps pass the time, and is a chance to socialize. In some cases, illness may interfere with a person's ability to enjoy or even tolerate food. If the doctor has not prescribed a special diet for your loved one, it is best to provide the foods that he or she normally eats.

Adequate fluid intake is also an important part of a healthy diet. Most people should drink at least eight 8-ounces glasses of fluid, every day. Fluids may include water, milk, juice, broth, or caffeine-free coffee, tea, or soft drinks. In some cases, such as for a person who has congestive heart failure, the doctor will limit the amount of fluids taken in each day. In such situations, it is especially important to carefully follow the doctor's instructions.

The following tips can help you help your loved one maintain a healthful diet. Adapt them to your specific needs and situation:

- Slice, dice, chop, mash, or puree foods to make them easy to chew and swallow.

- Look for ways to add calories and nutrients to the diet of a person who is at risk for weight loss. For example, fortified milk shakes can be tasty and nutritious. Your doctor may recommend a liquid nutritional supplement with a consistency similar to that of a milk shake.

- People with decreased appetites may consume more calories by eating five or six smaller meals throughout the day, rather than three large meals. Also, consider leaving healthy snacks, such as fresh fruit, carrots, and celery sticks, on the person's bedside table.

- Prepare your loved one's favorite foods. Ask what foods he or she likes and what he or she dislikes.

- Make meals look attractive. Be creative.

- Eat meals together whenever possible. Mealtime rituals can be comforting and can help restore a sense of normality to a person's life.

- If a stroke has paralyzed one side of a person's body, food may tend to collect in the paralyzed cheek. If this happens, gently knead the cheek with your finger while the person is chewing, to help move the food along.

- Whenever possible, encourage and help the person to exercise. Exercise stimulates the appetite and helps prevent constipation. Also, regular exercise, even when a person is confined to bed or a wheelchair, can stimulate the circulation and help maintain muscle tone. Your loved one may be able to perform simple weight lifting, stretching, and range-of-motion exercises with or without your assistance. Ask your doctor which exercises are best.

Chewing and Swallowing

Proper mouth care is essential for maintaining a healthy diet. Chewing and swallowing food may be difficult or impossible if a person has oral problems such as mouth sores, cavities, poorly fitting dentures, or untreated gum disease. Make sure that the person practices good oral hygiene (daily brushing and flossing) and that he or she has regular dental care.

If your loved one is unable to chew or swallow—because of oral radiation treatments, jaw injury, or stroke, for example—you may need to provide nutrition using an alternate method such as tube feeding or intravenous (directly into a vein) feeding. In such cases, it is extremely important to work closely with a healthcare professional to ensure that you know how to perform the method correctly and safely while causing the person the least amount of discomfort. Whenever you use an alternate feeding method, it is important to watch closely for any signs of infection, such as pain, redness, swelling at the insertion site of the intravenous needle or feeding tube, or fever.

If your loved one cannot feed himself or herself, you must do it for him or her. Cut food into small, bite-size pieces or puree it to make it easy to chew and swallow. Before feeding your loved one, be sure he or she is sitting upright in a comfortable position, and tuck a napkin or hand towel under his or her chin to catch any spills. Taste the food to be sure it is not too hot. Because feeding someone often is a lengthy process, put the food in a warming dish to keep it warm.

Special Diets

If your loved one needs to follow a special diet, your doctor can refer you to a nurse or registered dietitian who can provide you with detailed information about the particular diet. A registered dietitian can assess the person's dietary needs, provide guidance, and answer any questions you may have about the diet. Cookbooks are available for most special diets. Ask your doctor or dietitian to recommend one.

People who are receiving chemotherapy, radiation therapy, or other anticancer treatments may have special needs regarding diet and nutrition. These treatments often cause nausea and vomiting, which may be relieved with prescription medications. Discuss this possibility with your doctor if your loved one is having problems digesting foods and fluids.

Low-Sodium Diet

You can usually reduce the amount of sodium in a person's diet by not adding salt to food when you cook or serve it. To maintain a low-sodium diet, it is also important to avoid foods that are high in sodium, such as cured or tenderized meat (including ham, bacon, and cold cuts), smoked fish or meat, cheese, pickles, canned foods other than fruit, processed and prepared foods, and salted butter or margarine. Always check package labels for the sodium content of canned, prepared, and processed foods.

If you need to further restrict your loved one's salt intake, your doctor can tell you how to cut down on or eliminate foods that contain even small amounts of sodium. To add flavor to foods without adding salt, season them with spices, herbs, or lemon juice. Ask your doctor if it is appropriate to use a salt substitute. Most people find that after several salt-free weeks, they do not miss it.

Low-Protein Diet

Reducing the amount of protein in the diet involves cutting down on protein-rich foods such as eggs, meat, fish, and dairy products. Because protein supplies a significant portion of the body's energy requirements, you will need to compensate by adding extra fat and sugar to the diet. If your loved one needs to cut back on protein, ask your doctor or dietitian for guidance.

Liquid Diet

Sometimes a doctor will prescribe a liquid diet when the person cannot eat any solid food. In this case, your doctor can refer you to a dietitian who can plan an appropriately balanced diet. Also, you may want to ask your doctor about giving the person liquid nutritional supplements, which are widely available in single-serving cans.

When giving liquids, always elevate the person's head slightly to help prevent choking and spilling. The best way to do this is to hold the cup or glass while the person drinks through a flexible drinking straw.

Pressure Sores

Many people who require home care are confined to bed, posing a number of challenges for the person and his or her caregiver. Pressure sores, or bedsores, are one of the most common problems for people who are confined to bed. Pressure sores develop when certain areas of the body become compressed, either from remaining in the same position for long periods or because of prolonged contact with devices such as splints or casts. These painful sores can develop quickly and can become infected; in severe cases, hospitalization may be necessary.

The following conditions can put a person at increased risk of developing pressure sores:

- Immobility
- Incontinence
- Diabetes
- Poor circulation
- Being in traction or having splints or bandages
- Loss of sensation in specific areas of the body

Watch carefully for areas of the skin that become red, shiny, and insensitive to touch. When caught early, the sores can be treated by washing, applying lotions, using protective skin pads or shields, and repositioning the person at regular intervals to relieve pressure. If a pressure sore breaks open or begins to peel, call the doctor or nurse immediately. For additional information on pressure sores, see page 110.

Hygiene

Keeping the person you are caring for feeling clean and fresh is an important part of your job as a caregiver. Feeling clean can often help speed a person's recovery and boost his or her morale. Regular bathing can also help prevent pressure sores. Have the person wash his or her face and hands and brush his or her teeth at least twice a day.

Bathing

Unless a person is extremely ill, he or she can usually give himself or herself at least a sponge bath. Before bringing the person a basin of warm water, mild soap, and a washcloth for a sponge bath, place a large towel under him or her to protect the bedding. Provide another large towel to drape over the person for warmth and privacy, and make sure that the room is warm. He or she should have a sponge bath once a day.

If your loved one is unable to bathe, you can give him or her a bath in bed. Although giving a bed bath presents challenges, it is not a difficult task to perform once you have mastered the routine. Make sure that the room is warm before undressing the person, taking care to provide as much privacy as possible. Cover him or her with a large towel and place another towel underneath to protect the bedding. If the person is immobile or difficult to move, place the bottom towel into position as you would to change a bottom sheet (see page 26). Before you begin, check the water to make sure it is at a comfortable temperature. Use a mild soap that will not dry out or irritate the person's skin.

As you bathe the person, look carefully for sores, rashes, or other skin problems. If your loved one is recovering from surgery, be sure to examine the incision carefully to make sure that it is healing properly. Some indications of possible infection include fever; redness, pain, and swelling around the incision; and greenish or yellowish foul-smelling drainage. It is important to report any of these signs to the doctor or nurse immediately.

Follow these steps for giving a bath in bed:

STEP 1. Wash and dry one area of the person's body at a time, uncovering only the part of the body you are washing. This helps keep the person warm and maintains a sense of privacy.

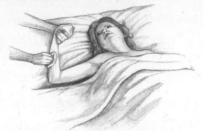

STEP 2. Bathe the person starting from the head down. Use soap only in sweaty areas, such as the armpits, groin, and buttocks. Be thorough but gentle. Change the water as needed.

STEP 3. Gently pat the person dry with a fresh, soft towel—do not rub.

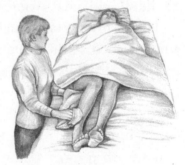

STEP 4. Roll the person onto one side to wash and dry his or her back.

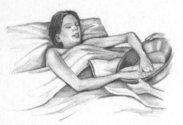

STEP 5. Let the person dip his or her hands into a basin of fresh water. This is more refreshing than having the hands wiped with a washcloth.

STEP 6. Before helping the person dress, make sure every area of his or her body is thoroughly dry. Provide or apply deodorant, lotion, or body powder as needed.

Washing Hair

Having clean hair also contributes to a person's sense of well-being. Even when someone is confined to bed, it is possible to wash his or her hair. To keep the bedding dry, place a vinyl sheet under a towel beneath the person's head, neck, and shoulders. Move the person down the bed, raise his or her shoulders on a pillow, and place a dishpan or a basin specially designed for this purpose under his or her head.

Wet the hair before shampooing and rinse it afterward by pouring several cups of warm, clear water over it. For longer hair, rest the person's head over the edge of the bed, so that the hair hangs over a bowl or basin placed on the floor. Put one end of a large tray under the person's head and neck and the other end in the dishpan or basin. The water can then run down the tray and into the dishpan or basin. Be sure that you rinse and dry the person's hair completely after washing. To dry the hair, rub it gently but thoroughly with a warm towel. Finish drying the hair with a blow dryer.

Shaving

Whenever possible, it is important for a man to continue his daily shaving routine when he is ill or confined to bed. Shaving will keep up his morale and help him feel clean and refreshed. Even if your loved one is confined to bed, he may still be able to shave himself. Place a basin of warm water, a towel, shaving supplies, and a small shaving mirror within easy reach on a tray or bedside table (you should hold the mirror). Help him sit up; place pillows behind his back for support. If possible, your loved one may feel more comfortable shaving while sitting on the edge of the bed or in a chair (see page 110). Have him wash his face with warm water immediately before shaving to soften the beard and make shaving easier.

If your loved one cannot shave himself, you (or a visiting nurse or trained home health aide) will need to do it for him. If you feel confident, you can shave him with shaving cream and a regular razor, but it may be safer and easier to use an electric razor. You can shave the person while he is sitting up or reclining. Use a firm but gentle touch; pressing down too firmly on the razor can cause cuts, nicks, and skin irritation. Always shave in the direction in which the hair grows; shaving "against the grain" can cause ingrown hairs and skin irritation. Use short strokes and be especially careful when shaving near the nose, ears, mouth, chin, and Adam's apple. Rinse the blade thoroughly after every few strokes to keep it from clogging or dragging. Wipe away any excess shaving cream on the face with a moist washcloth or towel. Apply a small amount of aftershave lotion or moisturizer, if desired, to help soothe the skin.

WARNING: To avoid potentially dangerous nicks and cuts, people with diabetes and those who are taking anticoagulant drugs (blood thinners) should always shave with an electric razor.

Toilet Needs

People who are confined to bed usually need assistance with eliminating waste. Both urinating and moving the bowels can be difficult for someone who cannot simply get up and use the bathroom. He or she may feel awkward and embarrassed, and illness or immobility may contribute to the problem. In any case, whether using a bedpan, handheld urinal, or commode, be sure the person always has complete privacy. And always keep toilet paper and moist towelettes within easy reach.

Using a Commode

If the person is allowed to get out of bed for brief periods, using a bedside commode may be easiest. Help the person get out of bed (see page 110), onto the commode, and back into bed. After each use, remove the bedpan from the commode and empty it into the toilet, rinse it out, clean it thoroughly with a household disinfectant diluted with water, and return it to the commode.

Using a Bedpan

A person who is confined to bed will need to use a bedpan. A male will also need to use a handheld urinal. Your loved one may be reluctant to ask for the bedpan so you should ask frequently if he or she needs to use it. Because using a bedpan is awkward for most people, be sure to give the person complete privacy and plenty of time. Never rush someone who is using a bedpan; patience on your part is very important. Keeping this in mind can contribute to a faster recovery and help avoid problems such as constipation and fecal impaction (accumulation of hardened feces in the rectum).

Before giving the person the bedpan, sprinkle a small amount of body powder on the rim to make it easier to slip it under his or her buttocks. If the person cannot lift himself or herself onto the bedpan, he or she can use it while lying down. Lift the person's hips while another caregiver places the bedpan beneath the person's buttocks, with the open end toward the person's feet. If another caregiver is not available, the easiest way to place an immobile person on a bedpan is to turn him or her to one side, gently press the bedpan against his or her buttocks, press the bedpan firmly down into the mattress, and roll the person back on top of it. When he or she is finished, hold the bedpan firmly in place and roll him or her off it, away from you. Then make sure that the genital and rectal areas are thoroughly cleaned and dried.

After each use, empty the bedpan and handheld urinal into the toilet, rinse them, wash them thoroughly with a household disinfectant diluted with water, and return them to the same place so that you can find them quickly when needed. Always leave a handheld urinal within easy reach so that the person does not have to ask for it. Keeping it in a large bowl or bucket will help to prevent spills.

Some caregivers may have to monitor a catheter or give enemas. To learn to perform these tasks effectively, you will need clear, precise instructions and the assistance of a healthcare professional, such as a nurse.

Symptoms to Monitor

As your loved one's caregiver, you are in the best position to observe any changes in his or her condition that may indicate an improvement or decline in health. What you watch for depends in large part on the person's particular illness or injury. In general, it is important to evaluate regularly your loved one's alertness, memory, mobility, vision, hearing, emotions, sleeping patterns, eating habits, personal interactions, and sensory responses such as touch. Even small, apparently insignificant changes can indicate a serious underlying health problem and should be reported to your doctor or nurse as soon as possible. Common signs to watch for include:

- Changes in breathing patterns, including shallow breathing, hyperventilation (abnormally deep, rapid, or prolonged breathing), raspy breathing, gurgling noises in the throat, temporary cessation of breathing (including during sleep), difficulty breathing, or wheezing
- Changes in mobility, such as limping, problems maintaining balance, restricted use of arms or legs, or paralysis
- Tremors, shaking, facial tics, twitching, drooping eyelids or mouth, or facial paralysis
- Unusual sneezing or coughing
- Discharge, such as through a bandage; a bloody nose or leaking eye; or pus oozing through an open sore
- Fever, chills, or sweating

- Insomnia (difficulty falling asleep or staying asleep) or fatigue
- Constipation, diarrhea, loss of bladder or bowel control, or vomiting
- Changes in urine or stool, including frequency, smell, appearance, and quantity, and pain or difficulty urinating or moving the bowels
- Changes in skin appearance, including rashes, sores, tenderness, dryness, moistness, itchiness, paleness, jaundice (yellowing of the skin and whites of the eyes), or swelling
- Unexplained weight loss or gain
- Changes in appetite

Depression

Identifying depression in older people can be difficult, and it is not uncommon for doctors and caregivers to mistake the symptoms of depression for another illness or for dementia. Even when depression is correctly diagnosed, an older person may not receive proper treatment. Some people mistakenly believe that depression is a normal part of aging rather than a treatable illness. If you notice that your loved one has any of the following signs or symptoms that persist for more than a few days, talk to his or her doctor immediately:

- Changes in mood or emotions
- Lack of responsiveness or attentiveness
- Lack of interest in his or her surroundings or things that were formerly pleasurable
- Feelings of hopelessness or helplessness

It is essential to have the doctor evaluate your loved one. If the diagnosis is depression, the doctor may prescribe medication or counseling, or both. The majority of cases of depression can be treated successfully at any age.

Fever

Although a fever is not necessarily dangerous, you should always notify the doctor whenever your loved one has a fever. Never try to have him or her "sweat out" a fever by turning up the heat or putting on extra blankets. This could raise the person's temperature even higher. Be sure to talk to your doctor before giving aspirin or an aspirin substitute to help bring down a fever.

 WARNING: Do not give aspirin to a child or adolescent who is ill with a fever; use of aspirin in children has been linked with Reye's syndrome, a potentially fatal condition.

If your loved one's temperature continues to rise after he or she has been given medication to reduce it, call your doctor immediately. In the meantime, relieve his or her discomfort by sponging his or her face, neck, arms, and legs with lukewarm water. Let the body dry naturally (evaporation cools the skin). While the temperature is falling, the person may sweat a lot. Be sure to encourage him or her to drink plenty of water, fruit juice, and broth to help replace body fluids and sodium lost through sweating.

Vomiting

Illness, medication, and various treatments, such as radiation therapy, may cause nausea and vomiting. Although some vomiting can be expected in such circumstances, frequent vomiting may be a sign of an underlying health problem. Talk to your doctor or nurse if vomiting persists.

If your loved one is confined to bed or cannot get to the bathroom quickly, leave a bowl, dishpan, or other suitable container at the bedside. The person may want to be left alone while vomiting, or may find it comforting to have you hold his or her forehead for support. After the person has vomited, offer some water to rinse the mouth and a bowl to spit into, then gently sponge his or her face with cool or lukewarm water.

After an episode of vomiting, do not give the person solid food for several hours, but as soon as the nausea ends, give sips of clear liquids such as water, tea, ginger ale, or broth to replace lost body fluids. Let the person decide the type of liquid he or she can drink. Soft, bland foods such as boiled potatoes, oatmeal, and gelatin may be easier to eat at this time.

If the person vomits repeatedly, call your doctor for advice. The doctor may recommend that you watch the person for signs of dehydration, including thirst, dry lips and mouth, dizziness, headache, confusion, muscle weakness, shakiness, and reduced output of urine. Dehydration is a potentially dangerous condition that, if not treated, can lead to coma and death.

Bed Making

Make the bed once a day and straighten it as needed. Change the sheets at least every 4 or 5 days, or whenever they become soiled. Use 100-percent cotton sheets, to absorb sweat. Always pull the bottom sheet taut to eliminate wrinkles, and tuck it in well. Arrange the pillows so that they support the person's shoulders and head. The best arrangement is to place two pillows side by side vertically against the headboard, and a third pillow across their base (see illustration).

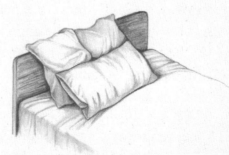

If the person prefers one pillow, place it low enough so that his or her head, neck, and shoulders are supported comfortably. A person who can sit upright needs greater support for his or her back. Provide this by adding more pillows or by using a lounging pillow with armrests.

To keep a shorter person from sliding toward the foot of the bed, provide something to brace the feet, such as a cushion or rolled-up blanket (see illustration).

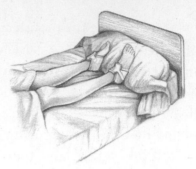

Changing a Bottom Sheet

It is possible to change the sheets even when the person you are caring for cannot get out of bed. To change a bottom sheet, follow these step-by-step instructions:

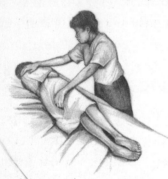

STEP 1. Slowly and carefully roll the person onto his or her side.

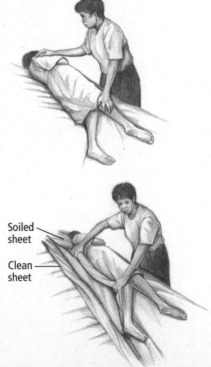

STEP 2. Gently move the person toward you, near the edge of the bed, making sure that he or she is lying in a stable position.

STEP 3. Roll half of the soiled sheet lengthwise against the person's back. Roll half of the clean sheet lengthwise and put it on the bed with the rolled half of the sheet down the center of the bed and the other half on the empty side of the bed.

Soiled sheet

Clean sheet

STEP 4. Carefully roll the person onto the flat, clean half and take off the soiled sheet. Unroll the rest of the clean sheet, stretch it tight, and tuck it in.

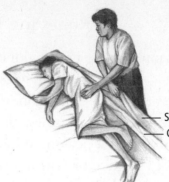

— Soiled sheet
— Clean sheet

Drawsheets

A drawsheet is an ordinary flat sheet that is folded and positioned in such a way as to provide a clean, unwrinkled bottom sheet without having to remake the bed. Fold the sheet in half lengthwise and put it over the bed crosswise, so that it extends from the person's head to his or her knees, and overlaps the bed more on one side than the other. Tuck in one end, pull the sheet tight, and tuck in the other end. When you want to provide a clean surface, untuck both ends of the sheet, pull a clean area from the longer end into position, and tuck in both ends tightly again. For comfort, make sure that the drawsheet is pulled tight to each side and free of wrinkles.

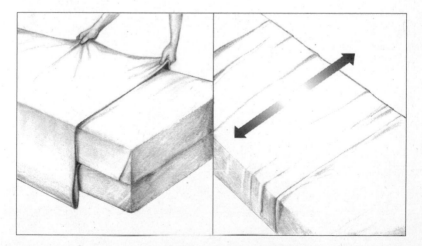

You can also use a drawsheet to move an immobile person up in bed and to turn him or her from side to side (see page 115).

Relieving Boredom

Many people like to be left alone to rest when they are ill. Others prefer to have company or some type of entertainment to help pass the time. Television, videos, radio, a computer, reading material, games, puzzles, and the company of other people can help occupy a person's mind and ease boredom or frustration. Ask your doctor how much the person can reasonably do and encourage him or her to engage in as many enjoyable activities as possible.

3

Specialized
Caregiving Skills

In some cases, a person's needs or situation requires the expertise and training of a registered nurse or other professional caregiver. But with proper training and guidance, most home caregivers can learn to perform these tasks.

Wound Care

Caring for a wound requires both skill and patience. If your loved one is returning home from the hospital with an open wound, ask a nurse in the hospital to teach both of you how to care for the wound before discharge. The nurse, social worker, or doctor will probably also refer your loved one to a home healthcare agency for follow-up care. This helps to ensure that proper procedures are followed and reduces the risk of complications, such as infection. If a doctor is monitoring the wound, he or she will refer your loved one for follow-up home care so that a trained healthcare professional can supervise care of the wound.

Wet-to-Dry Saline Dressings

The most common type of wound care consists of applying wet-to-dry saline dressings. Saline is a saltwater solution that you can find at drugstores and medical supply companies. Ask your doctor or nurse to recommend one. With wet-to-dry dressings, the layer of gauze closest to the wound is wet, with subsequent layers of dry gauze over that layer. This type of dressing ensures that the healing tissue remains clean and moist, which helps the wound to heal. Germs cannot reach the wound because of the multiple layers of dry gauze over the moist layer. You should change the dressing at least once a day, and often up to three or four times a day, depending on the amount of drainage from the wound and the recommendation of the doctor.

How to Change a Dressing

Before changing a dressing, wash your hands thoroughly (for at least one minute) with soap and water. Use liquid soap because it provides less opportunity for bacteria to grow. (Bacteria can grow on the surface of bar soap or in a soap dish.) Assemble all of the equipment you need before removing the old dressing. Wear disposable latex gloves throughout the process to avoid contaminating the wound and to protect yourself from infection.

STEP 1.   Remove the tape that holds the old dressing in place and lift the old dressing from the wound. Do this gently and carefully, because the old dressing may be dry and firmly attached to the wound.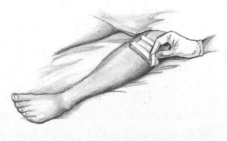

If this occurs, moisten the old dressing with saline solution to soften it and make it easier to remove.

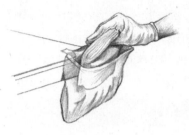

STEP 2. Place the old dressing in a sealable plastic bag, then seal the bag and throw it in the trash. Remove your latex gloves and carefully discard them. Before cleaning the wound, put on a fresh pair of gloves, being careful not to touch the wound.

STEP 3. Use sterile gauze pads to carefully clean the wound with saline or a commercial solution designed to disinfect the area and promote new tissue formation. (Use

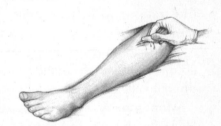

the solution the doctor has prescribed or recommended.) Holding all four corners of the pad, wipe the wound firmly but gently with the untouched portion of the pad. You may need to use more than one pad. Carefully discard the used gauze pads.

STEP 4. Open the new dressing packet and pour the saline or other solution sparingly onto the gauze. Apply enough solution to wet the gauze without soaking it. Place the new dressing over the wound. (The number of

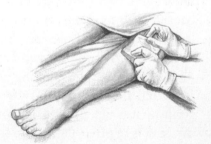

gauze pads needed to cover the wound will depend on the size of the wound.) Place one or more dry sterile pads over the wet one and secure them with tape. Use paper tape because it is less irritating to the skin. (Paper tape is available at drugstores and medical supply companies.)

Some doctors prescribe antibiotic creams for wounds that are not healing properly. After the wound has been cleaned with the appropriate solution, you can apply the cream to the open wound with a sterile gauze pad. In this situation, you should not

Montgomery Straps

If you are changing dressings frequently and the person's skin is getting sore beneath the tape, try using Montgomery straps (see illustration) to help prevent the irritation of frequent tape removal. You can leave Montgomery straps on the skin for up to 5 days (or as long as the person can tolerate them) and still be able to make frequent dressing changes.

Montgomery straps are backed with tape. To apply Montgomery straps, tape the straps to the person's skin on either side of the wound and flatten them until they meet in the middle of the gauze covering the wound. (The portion of the straps covering the gauze is also backed with tape but will not stick to the wound.) Each strap has several round holes on the edge. Lace string through the holes to tie the straps together and firmly hold the dressing in place. To change the dressing, simply untie the straps and carefully fold them back from the wound, leaving the part of the straps that is taped to the person's skin in place. When the new dressing is in place, flatten the straps over the gauze covering the wound and retie them. A nurse will teach you how to correctly apply and remove Montgomery straps.

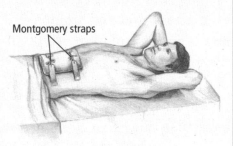

Montgomery straps

use a wet-to-dry saline dressing because it would decrease the effectiveness of the antibiotic cream. Ask your doctor or nurse for advice.

⚠ **WARNING:** Never apply hydrogen peroxide or iodine solution to an open wound. These substances are toxic to the cells of a wound that is healing. Use only the solution that the doctor has prescribed.

Other Types of Wound Dressings

A variety of newer dressing materials are available that offer more flexibility than the standard wet-to-dry dressings. These dressings include algae, colloidal compositions, transparent films, polyurethane foams, granules, and absorbent sheets. All of these materials can absorb drainage from a wound, hold the drainage in place until the dressing is changed, and keep the wound clean. The presence of drainage actually helps the wound heal and promotes growth of new tissue.

Although these dressings are different from the standard wet-to-dry saline dressings, the technique for changing them is basically the same: remove the old dressing, clean the wound with saline or a prescribed solution, and cover the wound with a new dressing. You still use two pairs of latex gloves—one to remove the old dressing and the other to apply the new one. Make sure that the wound does not close at the surface before new tissue has filled in the depth of the wound. If the top of the wound heals first, it can trap drainage and dead tissue, and an abscess can develop. If this occurs, a doctor or nurse may have to reopen the top layer of the wound to promote proper healing.

Wound Infection

Occasionally, a wound may become infected. You can recognize an infection by the color and smell of the drainage and the redness of the tissue surrounding the wound. In an infection, the drainage may increase, be green or yellow and tinged with blood, or it may have a foul odor. The person may have a fever. He or she may also have significant pain. Call the doctor right away if this occurs. He or she may recommend a different type of dressing or solution, or alter the frequency of dressing changes. He or she may prescribe antibiotics to fight the infection. If there is dead tissue at the site of the wound, the doctor may scrape it away to allow new, healthy tissue to grow.

Incontinence

Incontinence, the inability to control the passage of urine (urinary incontinence) or stool (fecal incontinence), is usually caused by an underlying disease or condition. Urinary and fecal incontinence can occur separately or together. Do not accept incontinence as a normal part of aging. An older person who is experiencing problems with incontinence should be examined as soon as possible by a doctor.

Incontinence can be a major problem when caring for a loved one at home. One way to deal with incontinence is to establish a toilet routine: encourage the person to use the toilet at frequent, regular intervals (for example, every 2 to 3 hours). Provide any necessary assistance promptly, to prevent accidents.

Make sure that the toilet facilities are readily accessible and easy to use, with handrails in place alongside the toilet, if possible. Provide night-lights in hallways and in the bathroom. For a person who has memory problems, it may also be helpful to provide signs guiding the way to the bathroom, with a sign that reads BATHROOM attached to the bathroom door. If the person is confined to bed, make sure that a commode (a portable chair that contains a removable bedpan) or bedpan and handheld urinal are within easy reach.

If the person is unable to wipe after urinating or having a bowel movement, you will need to do it for him or her. Keeping the genital and rectal areas clean is important for helping to prevent skin problems. Always wipe a female gently from front to back (from the vagina to the rectum) to ensure that fecal matter does not enter the vagina or urinary tract and cause infection.

A number of incontinence aids, such as absorbent incontinence pads, disposable briefs, and condom catheters, are available from drugstores and medical supply companies. Ask your doctor about using them. In some difficult cases of urinary incontinence, an indwelling catheter (a plastic tube inserted into the bladder that drains urine into a bag) may be used. The bag needs to be emptied and cleaned regularly. Your doctor, a visiting nurse, or other trained healthcare professional will change the catheter periodically.

When someone develops both urinary and fecal incontinence, loss of bladder control usually occurs before loss of bowel control. Before making any changes in the day-to-day management of incontinence, the doctor will examine the person to find the underlying cause. This, in turn, will help the doctor determine the best course of treatment.

Urinary Incontinence

Urinary tract infections can often cause sudden-onset, or acute, incontinence. In such cases, once the infection has been treated successfully, the incontinence stops. The use of diuretics (medications that increase the body's output of water) can also lead to urinary incontinence. If diuretics are prescribed for your loved one, make sure that you give them early in the morning to avoid having his or her bladder fill at night during sleep. Some other medications can also cause bladder-control problems. For example, medications such as sleeping pills and tranquilizers can reduce a person's ability to react to bladder sensations and get to the bathroom quickly. Your doctor may decide to change medications or adjust the dosage to help control the problem.

Other possible causes of urinary incontinence are consuming large amounts of caffeine (found in coffee, tea, and colas) or drinking a lot of alcohol. Switching to caffeine-free beverages and avoiding alcohol (especially in the evening before bedtime) can help reduce urinary incontinence.

Dehydration (abnormally low levels of water in body tissues) can cause a person's urine to become concentrated, which, in turn, can irritate the bladder outlet muscles and result in loss of bladder control. The best way to prevent dehydration is to increase the intake of fluids. Have your loved one drink at least eight glasses (8 ounces each) of fluid every day. Fluids may include water, milk, juice, broth, and caffeine-free coffee, tea, and soft drinks. Increased fluid volume in the body decreases urine concentration, thereby decreasing the risk of bladder irritation.

Urinary incontinence sometimes accompanies diseases or conditions such as diabetes, heart failure, or prostate problems. Some neurologic (brain and nervous system) problems, such as stroke and Alzheimer's disease, can also cause bladder-control problems. These medical conditions must be treated before the incontinence can be controlled. If your loved one has incontinence, he or she should see a doctor promptly for an examination.

Dealing with Urinary Incontinence

Many older people are embarrassed by incontinence and may try to hide the problem from relatives and friends. If you have noticed any possible signs of incontinence (such as underwear soaking in the bathroom sink, stains in underwear or clothing in the laundry, or the smell of urine on chair cushions), use care and sensitivity in approaching the person about it. Avoid making an accusation, which could cause him or her to refuse the necessary medical examination and treatment because of embarrassment and denial.

There are more effective ways to help a person deal with urinary incontinence. For example, reminding the person to use the bathroom at least every 2 hours during the day can help ensure that his or her bladder is emptied before it reaches the point at which it empties itself. Limit the person's intake of fluids after dinner and before bedtime and make sure that he or she goes to the bathroom immediately before going to bed. Have a handheld urinal available for a man who cannot get to the bathroom quickly or who is confined to bed. Have a bedpan available for a woman in the same situation; attempt to assist her to an upright position on the bedpan so that she is sitting in the normal position for urination. Consider providing a bedside commode for any person who has difficulty getting to the bathroom quickly but who can get in and out of bed on his or her own.

Absorbent disposable briefs can help protect clothing, bedding, mattresses, and furniture. You may want to try several different brands to determine which one best suits the needs of your loved one. You might be able to save money by purchasing your favorite brand in bulk from a medical supply company. In any case, to preserve your loved one's dignity and to avoid embarrassment, always refer to the pads as adult briefs or disposable briefs. Never refer to them as diapers.

Change the pads as soon as they become soiled. Wearing a soiled pad for any period of time can cause skin irritation and lead to the development of pressure sores; it can also make a person feel ashamed and embarrassed. A person who uses incontinence pads or wears disposable briefs should use the toilet every 2 hours during the day. Ideally, he or she should wear loose-fitting, washable clothing. Clothes with zippers, snaps, or Velcro are easiest to put on and remove.

If weakening of pelvic muscles is the cause of your loved one's urinary incontinence, have him or her perform exercises to strengthen the muscles and help improve bladder control. Give him or her the following instructions for these exercises, which are often referred to as Kegel exercises:

STEP 1.   Practice contracting (tightening) your pelvic-floor muscles by stopping and restarting the flow of urine midstream several times while you are urinating.

STEP 2.   Contract the muscles and hold for a count of 2 to 3 seconds at first, eventually working up to 8 to 10 seconds. The longer the contraction, the greater the benefit.

STEP 3.   Perform a set of 10 contractions at least five times a day, every day. You can perform these exercises in any position, anytime, anyplace. No one will know that you are exercising.

Urinary Catheter Care

Another challenge to the caregiver is managing an indwelling (inside-the-body) urinary catheter. A catheter is tubing made of rubber or synthetic material that is used to channel urine from the bladder into a collection bag outside the body. A catheter is inserted by a doctor or nurse and is used for a number of conditions or situations. For example, a catheter may be necessary if a person has problems urinating and the doctor is concerned that the bladder may not completely empty. A catheter can also be used to help prevent infection when a person has an open wound in the groin area.

An indwelling urinary catheter requires special attention because of the risk of infection. Always wash your hands with plenty of soap and hot water both before and after handling a urinary catheter. And always wear a fresh pair of disposable gloves. The tubing of the catheter enters the urethra, the channel through which urine passes from the bladder to outside the body. Use liquid soap and water to clean the area where the tubing enters the urethra. Rinse the area with clear water and gently dry it. You may also use a prepared disinfectant to clean the area if the doctor has prescribed or recommended one.

Before reconnecting the drainage tubing to the bag, clean the tubing with an alcohol pad or other skin disinfectant, such as povidone-iodine solution. Always position the urine collection bag below the level of the bladder to facilitate drainage of urine out of the bladder. This will also help prevent urine from backing up into the bladder and causing an infection.

The urine collection bag can usually collect up to 1 or 2 quarts of urine. However, be sure to check the bag frequently and empty it before it becomes full. The bottom of the collection bag has a valve to allow urine to drain into another container. Empty the bag at least once a day.

A visiting nurse must come to the home at regular intervals to change the catheter. In general, if the catheter is draining well, it should be changed approximately once a month. If sediment or mucus collects in the tubing, it can become blocked. A catheter should continually drain urine. If urine does not enter the bag for a period of approximately 2 hours, the tubing may be blocked, which can be serious. Contact the visiting nurse immediately. If you are not using the services of a visiting nurse, contact the doctor immediately; you may have to take the person to a hospital emergency department to have the blockage cleared.

Irrigating a Catheter   Some doctors recommend routine irrigation of a catheter (cleansing it by gently flushing it with an irrigating solution) to prevent clogging. A nurse can show you how to irrigate a catheter whenever it becomes clogged or is flowing slowly. Never try to irrigate a catheter unless you have been trained in how to do it.

If a catheter is clogged, the person may feel some pressure in the lower abdomen and urine may leak around the catheter onto bedding or incontinence pads. If this occurs, the catheter needs to be either changed or irrigated. If you have been trained, you can irrigate a catheter with a bulb syringe (a type of syringe that resembles a turkey baster). Disconnect the catheter from the collection bag. Then remove the bulb and place the tip of the sterile syringe into the catheter (the tubing that goes directly into the person's bladder). Pour the irrigating solution slowly and carefully through the syringe and into the tubing to dislodge the sediment or blockage and allow urine to flow freely. If this does not work, have the visiting nurse come right away to change the catheter.

> **WARNING:** When a person has a urinary catheter, it is important to prevent bacteria from entering the urinary tract and causing an infection. To help prevent contamination when you disconnect the tubing from the catheter or the collection bag, be careful not to place the sterile ends of the tubing on an unsterile surface. Use alcohol or another skin disinfectant to clean the catheter and the tubing before reconnecting them.

How to Prevent a Catheter from Clogging

Here are some steps you can take to keep a catheter draining well and reduce the risk of infection:

- Have the person drink at least eight glasses (8 ounces each) of liquid (water or juice) every day.
- Give the person cranberry juice during the day to help make the urine more acidic, which may help prevent bacteria from collecting in the bladder.
- Keep the collection bag below the level of the bladder at all times to help prevent backup of urine.
- Keep all tubing straight and watch for kinks.
- Avoid placing the tubing under the person's leg because the weight of the leg can block the flow of urine.

Leg Bags   If a person who has a urinary catheter is able to leave the house but does not want to bring along a standard urine collection bag, he or she can use a leg bag instead. A leg bag is a small urine collection bag that is connected to the urinary catheter and strapped to the person's leg. This allows the bag to be hidden under clothing. The storage capacity of a leg bag is significantly less than that of a standard collection bag, but if emptied frequently, it can be both effective and inconspicuous. The visiting nurse can show you how to attach a leg bag.

Fecal Incontinence

Fecal incontinence can be more challenging for a caregiver than urinary incontinence. Though having to care for a person with fecal incontinence may sometimes make you feel stressed and angry, never scold the person for an accident or make him or her clean it up as a punishment.

Eating a healthy diet is one way to help promote normal bowel function. Make sure that your loved one eats plenty of high-fiber foods (such as fresh fruits, vegetables, and whole grains) and drinks plenty of fluids. If possible, keep track of when he or she usually has a bowel movement, and try to have him or her use the toilet at that time every day. Ask the doctor if you can use glycerin suppositories to stimulate bowel movements (the person will have a bowel movement within 15 to 20 minutes after insertion of the suppository). If fecal impaction (accumulation of hardened feces in the rectum) is the cause of the incontinence, a doctor or nurse must remove the impacted feces from the rectum.

Managing Intravenous Medications

Some people need intravenous therapy, which is the infusion of nutrients or medication directly into the bloodstream. In a home-care setting, this treatment is usually provided by a visiting nurse who has been trained to perform the procedure. For intravenous therapy, a needle is inserted into a vein, often (but not always) on the top of the hand, and a thin tube (catheter) is threaded into the vein. The needle is removed and an infusion device may be attached to the catheter to maintain access to the vein. The infusion device (often referred to as a heparin lock) is filled with diluted heparin, an anticoagulant drug that prevents blood clots from forming in the tubing.

After the catheter is securely inserted in the person's vein, the nurse will begin giving the medication, showing you how to handle the tubing and the intravenous solution. If you are willing and able, the nurse may also teach you how to do the actual infusion. He or she may return once a day (or as often as needed) to change the intravenous catheter. The nurse will do this only after he or she is certain that you can safely and confidently perform the procedure and handle the equipment.

A delivery service or the visiting nurse will bring the solutions or medications the doctor prescribes to the person's home. Many intravenous solutions must be stored in the refrigerator. Before giving any refrigerated medication intravenously, remove it from the refrigerator and let it stand at room temperature for about half an hour. Right before you attach the tubing with solution to the intravenous catheter, flush the catheter with saline solution, heparin, or both. (The nurse will show you how to do this as a part of managing the tubing.) Flushing the catheter will ensure that the line is unobstructed, free of clots, and that the solution will flow freely. Flush the intravenous line again immediately after the infusion to keep it unobstructed.

Depending on the site of insertion and the device used to measure out the solution, the person may be able to walk around while receiving intravenous therapy. Some solutions are administered by gravity drainage, in which the bag containing the solution is at a higher level than the site of insertion. The bag is usually connected to an intravenous pole that can be adjusted to the appropriate height. The solution must always remain hanging or connected to the intravenous pole. The solution flows at a set rate. Tell the nurse immediately about any change you notice in the rate of flow.

> **NOTE:** Be sure that a person who is receiving intravenous therapy does not pull at the insertion site or the attached tubing. If the tubing becomes twisted or kinked, carefully straighten it, making sure that the catheter remains in place and the tubing stays attached.

Complications of Intravenous Therapy

Intravenous therapy can cause complications, such as inflammation of the vein that is being used for the therapy. Symptoms of inflammation include redness and tenderness at the tip of the catheter and along the vein, a puffy area over the vein, and fever. Report these symptoms to your doctor or nurse immediately.

Another possible complication of intravenous therapy is infiltration of the intravenous fluid into the surrounding tissue. This can occur if the catheter becomes dislodged from or passes through the vein. Symptoms include swelling, pain, a burning sensation, or a feeling of tightness around the insertion site. If this occurs, stop the infusion and contact the doctor or nurse immediately.

Another possible complication of intravenous therapy is a blocked intravenous line, which can interrupt the flow of fluid through the tubing. You can fix this problem by gently flushing the tubing with heparin. If this does not help, call the nurse immediately for assistance.

Risks of Immobility

Many people who are confined to bed develop problems related to immobility, which is a significant complication of many major illnesses. Immobility reduces lung function and heart output, increasing a person's risk of developing problems such as pneumonia and blood clots. A person who is confined to bed for longer than a day begins to lose strength. After one week in bed, he or she may be too weak to stand up unassisted. Because of these potential risks, a person who is able to get out of bed needs to do so on a regular basis.

Heart rate, or pulse, is a good indicator of how well a person's cardiovascular system can handle being out of bed. To check a person's heart rate, place your index and middle fingers along the carotid artery at the side of the neck or on the inside of his or her wrist (see illustrations). Do not use your thumb. You should be able to feel blood pulsing in the artery as the heart beats. To get the number of beats that occur in 1 minute, count the number of beats you can feel in exactly 15 seconds and multiply the number by four. This is the person's heart rate.

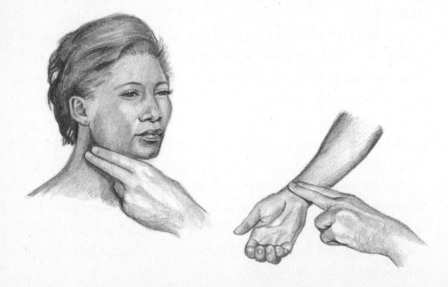

If the person's heart rate is between 50 and 100 beats per minute when out of bed and sitting in a chair, encourage him or her to stay up as long as possible. However, if the person's heart rate is higher than 100 beats per minute when he or she is calmly sitting in a chair, sitting up may be too strenuous and you need to help him or her back into bed. In this case, you should help the person perform some simple exercises in bed regularly to help increase his or her strength and endurance enough to get out of bed. These simple exercises can include range-of-motion exercises (see page 113), turning from side to side in bed, and sitting on the edge of the bed for short periods of time. If the person's heart rate is below 50 beats per minute, contact the doctor as soon as possible. A heart rate this low could indicate problems such as dehydration, anemia, or heart failure.

Respiratory Function

It's important for a person who is confined to bed to maintain respiratory function. Encourage the person to do deep-breathing exercises and cough to expand his or her lungs and help prevent pneumonia. Deep breathing and coughing should be done every hour during waking hours using a device called a spirometer to measure air expulsion. A home-care respiratory therapist can supply you with a spirometer and train you to use it. If you cannot get a spirometer or do not have the services of a respiratory therapist, simply encourage the person to breathe in through the nose as deeply as possible and then very slowly but forcibly breathe out through the mouth.

If the person develops symptoms including coughing, difficulty breathing, sputum that is green, gray, yellow, or brown, or fever, he or she may have pneumonia. If you notice these symptoms, contact the doctor immediately.

Deep Vein Thrombosis

Blood clots are another possible complication of immobility. They usually develop in the deep or superficial (near the surface) veins of the legs. If the person is unable to bear weight or walk, moving the legs as much as possible while in bed can help prevent blood clots. Also, ask the doctor about using special elastic stockings that help prevent blood clots from forming in the legs.

WARNING: Never massage an immobile person's legs, especially the calves, because doing so can dislodge a clot that has already developed. The clot can travel through the bloodstream to the lungs, causing blockage of an artery that supplies blood to the lungs (pulmonary embolism). Symptoms of pulmonary embolism include sudden difficulty breathing, pain in the chest, rapid pulse, sweating, slight fever, productive cough (a cough that produces sputum), and blood in the sputum. This condition is a medical emergency. If these symptoms occur, call 911 or your local emergency number, or take the person to the nearest hospital emergency department without delay.

Dealing with Specific Illnesses

Different illnesses require different levels and types of care. For example, a person who has had a stroke may need physical therapy, while a person with diabetes may need help monitoring medications and diet. This section provides advice for caregivers on dealing with several common illnesses and conditions.

Influenza and Pneumonia

Influenza, or the flu, is a highly contagious respiratory infection that is caused by a virus. Influenza can be especially serious in young children, people with chronic diseases (such as heart disease, diabetes, or AIDS), people who are disabled, and older people. Flu symptoms include fever (between 101 and 104 degrees Fahrenheit), chills, headache, muscle pain, weakness, cough, runny nose, and swollen lymph glands in the neck. Treatment usually consists of bed rest, reducing the fever with a medication such as acetaminophen, drinking plenty of fluids (at least eight glasses daily, 8 ounces each), and taking cough syrup to relieve the cough and enable the person to sleep. Warm baths may help to relieve muscle pain. For safety reasons, many doctors recommend against using a heating pad to relieve muscle pain.

WARNING: If you use a heating pad to relieve muscle pain, always keep it set at "low" to reduce the risk of burns and skin damage. Always turn off the heating pad when it is not in use. Never go to sleep while using a heating pad, and do not use one overnight. Closely monitor all heating pad use, especially when caring for a person who is older, disabled, or immobile, or who has reduced sensation and cannot feel pain or heat.

Preventing the Flu from Spreading

Influenza can be spread very easily. Here are some helpful tips to help keep influenza from spreading:

- Wash your hands. Hand washing is the single most important step you can take to avoid spreading the flu virus from person to person. Make sure that everyone in the household, including the person who is receiving care, frequently washes his or her hands with plenty of soap and water.
- Discourage anyone with a respiratory infection from visiting.
- Dispose of all used tissues in a separate, closed container (a paper or plastic bag).

Get Your Shots

An annual flu shot at the beginning of the flu season—usually in October—is recommended for people with chronic diseases such as heart disease or diabetes, older people (age 65 and up), people receiving treatment for cancer, and people who are at high risk of exposure to the virus, such as healthcare workers. Because new strains of the virus develop each year, you need to get a flu shot every year. But you do not have to be in a high-risk group to benefit from a flu shot; immunization can reduce anyone's risk of developing the flu. However, if you are allergic or sensitive to eggs, you should not get a flu shot because the vaccine is made from eggs.

Check to make sure that the person you are caring for has been vaccinated against pneumococcal pneumonia, a common bacterial form of pneumonia. The vaccination is given once and is effective for life. Ask the doctor about these shots.

Watch carefully for any signs of complications from influenza, which can be more serious than the flu itself. Complications include pneumonia (either viral or bacterial) and worsening of a preexisting lung disease such as asthma, bronchitis, or emphysema. Common signs of pneumonia include a fever that lasts longer than 5 days accompanied by shortness of breath and coughing up of bloody or colored (green, gray, yellow, or brown) sputum.

If pneumonia develops, the doctor will treat it with antibiotics and may also prescribe nutrient supplements (if the person is unable to eat) and oxygen. Using acetaminophen instead of aspirin to reduce fever can help prevent Reye's syndrome, a rare but life-threatening condition linked to the use of aspirin in children and in people whose immune system has been weakened. A person who develops pneumonia after having the flu will be especially weak and may need many weeks to regain his or her strength. In some cases, depending on the person's age, the extent of the infection, and whether he or she also has a chronic condition (such as asthma or diabetes), the person may need to be hospitalized.

Diabetes

Diabetes is a disorder in which the body is unable to make or use glucose, a form of sugar that is the body's main source of energy. Many older people have diabetes, which can be treated effectively. A person with diabetes must closely follow a prescribed diet. Make sure you have clear instructions about your loved one's diet from his or her doctor or dietitian.

If the person is on insulin therapy, the doctor or nurse will give you clear instructions about coordinating the insulin with the person's intake of food. You will also be asked to monitor the person's blood glucose level to make sure that the insulin therapy is effective in keeping the glucose level in a healthy range. A daily fasting blood glucose test, performed using a drop of blood from the person's finger, can now be done easily at home using a portable machine called a glucometer. (Newer monitors are available that allow you to measure your blood glucose level without sticking your finger.)

A person with diabetes should always wear a medical alert bracelet or necklace that indicates that he or she has the condition. This helps ensure that proper medical treatment will be administered if he or she has a reaction called hypoglycemia (low blood sugar) while out. A reaction can occur if the diabetes medication (either insulin or oral medication) is not balanced by sufficient intake of food or if the person performs strenuous exercise without eating enough. Possible symptoms of hypoglycemia include headache, nervousness, hunger, dizziness, and feeling faint or fainting. A hypoglycemic reaction is serious; it can cause loss of consciousness and, if not treated quickly, can lead to severe, life-threatening complications. At the first sign of hypoglycemia, have the person eat a food that contains sugar, such as a piece of hard candy or half of a glass of orange juice. Then have him or her consume a longer-acting carbohydrate or protein such as a slice of bread or a glass of milk.

WARNING: To anticipate and treat a possible hypoglycemic reaction, anyone with diabetes who takes either oral hypoglycemic medication or insulin should always carry some food that contains sugar that the body can rapidly use. Glucose tablets, which provide quick relief from hypoglycemia, are available over-the-counter in drugstores.

People with diabetes are at increased risk of developing problems involving damage to the small blood vessels that move blood from the heart to body tissues. These complications include stroke, kidney disease, and heart attack. It is vital to strictly control blood sugar levels to help prevent these danger-ous complications.

Over time, diabetes can damage nerves and blood vessels in the feet. Small cuts can become infected and, if blood flow to the area is severely limited, can lead to gangrene (tissue death). In some cases, the toes need to be amputated to save the rest of the foot and leg. For this reason, you should never trim the toe-nails of a person with diabetes. Instead, take the person to a podiatrist (a specialist in diagnosing, treating, and preventing foot problems) for toenail trimming. Inspect the tops and soles of the person's feet daily, as well as the area between the toes, to look for signs of skin breakdown.

A person with diabetes should also have regular eye exami-nations performed by an ophthalmologist (a medical doctor who specializes in diseases of the eyes) to detect changes in the blood vessels in the eye. Without proper treatment, eye conditions related to diabetes can lead to vision problems such as diabetic retinopathy and blindness.

Angina

Angina is chest pain or pressure caused by an insufficient supply of oxygen to the heart muscle. Angina is usually the result of atherosclerosis, the formation of fatty deposits called plaques in the artery walls, which interferes with normal blood flow. In people with angina, the condition is often triggered by physical activity and lasts no more than a few minutes. Angina can also occur after eating a large meal or, in some cases, can come on at night while a person is resting or asleep. The first time it occurs, angina may be mistaken for a heart attack. But because a significant percentage of people with first-time angina may actually be having a heart attack, any new onset of angina should be treated as a medical emergency. If the person you are caring for has any pain or tightness in the chest, call 911 or your local emergency number or take him or her to the nearest hospital emergency department immediately.

In general, angina follows a unique pattern for each person. Any change in that pattern (such as changes in symptoms, intensity, or duration) must be immediately reported to the doctor. For example, if angina symptoms are usually brought on by exercise and now occur when the person is resting, this is a serious matter that requires immediate medical evaluation. Unstable angina (angina that occurs unpredictably or that suddenly increases in frequency or intensity) sometimes precedes a heart attack.

For many people, lifestyle changes can control or eliminate angina. If a person with angina smokes, he or she should quit immediately. If the person has a high cholesterol level, dietary changes or cholesterol-lowering medication can help bring it down. High blood pressure can be controlled with diet, exercise, and medication. Although exercise is good for people who have angina, it is extremely important to check with the doctor before beginning any type of exercise program. Talk to the doctor about the lifestyle changes your loved one needs to make. Once the doctor recommends appropriate changes, ask him or her for referrals to professionals who can help implement these changes—for example, a nutritionist or smoking-cessation counselor—or for helpful literature. Be patient and persistent when you encourage the person to make these difficult changes.

Even after making lifestyle changes, some people will need to take medication to control their angina. Nitroglycerin is the medication that is most often prescribed to treat this condition. This drug relaxes blood vessels, which increases the supply of blood and oxygen to the heart muscle and reduces its workload. Nitroglycerin is usually prescribed in pill form. One type of pill is placed under the tongue and allowed to dissolve; another type is swallowed whole. The drug also is available as an oral aerosol spray or as a time-release skin patch.

A person using the under-the-tongue form of nitroglycerin or an oral nitroglycerin spray to control angina should keep the medication nearby at all times so that he or she can take the drug as soon as symptoms occur. These forms of nitroglycerin can be taken before symptoms occur if the person knows that he or she will be participating in an activity that normally brings on an attack of angina. If the pain continues after taking nitroglycerin (after the pill has dissolved under the tongue), have the person take another pill in 5 minutes. If the second dose of nitroglycerin does not relieve the angina within 5 minutes, call 911 or your local emergency number or take the person immediately to the nearest hospital emergency department for treatment.

Other medications used to treat angina include beta-blockers and calcium channel blockers, both of which lower the heart rate and blood pressure and reduce the heart's demand for oxygen. Regardless of which medication the person is taking, be sure to carefully follow the doctor's instructions.

Heart Attack

A heart attack is the death of part of the heart muscle caused by sudden interruption of blood flow to that portion of the heart. Many people have symptoms—including worsening angina, shortness of breath, and unexplained fatigue—days and weeks ahead of a heart attack. Others, especially older people, may experience a "silent" heart attack in which the symptoms are so mild the heart attack goes undetected.

The symptoms of a heart attack include pain or pressure deep under the breastbone; the pain or pressure may radiate to the back, the left arm, or the neck and jaw. The pain may be similar to that of angina, but, unlike angina, the pain from a heart attack is rarely relieved by nitroglycerin or rest. The person's skin may be cool to the touch, but he or she may be sweating. He or she may be restless, apprehensive, pale, and nauseated, and may have indigestion. If nitroglycerin is available, have the person take some at this time, and call for emergency medical assistance immediately. It is safer to go to the nearest hospital emergency department right away than it is to wait and see if the pain stops. Because almost half of deaths from a heart attack occur within the first 3 to 4 hours, it is vital for anyone with symptoms to receive immediate emergency medical treatment.

If the person has no obvious pulse, is unconscious, is not breathing, and cannot be aroused, basic cardiopulmonary resuscitation (CPR) should be started *immediately* by someone who is trained in this lifesaving technique. Failure to begin resuscitation may result in the person's death. **All people caring for a person who has a history of heart disease need to learn the**

basic CPR techniques. The American Heart Association and the American Red Cross offer CPR classes in most communities; the classes usually are inexpensive or free.

Treatment for a heart attack consists of limiting the destruction of heart tissue, reducing the workload of the heart, relieving distress resulting from the symptoms, and preventing and treating complications that can arise from the loss of blood to the heart muscle. The person is hospitalized and usually confined to bed in the intensive care or coronary care unit for the first few days after a heart attack so that his or her condition can be closely monitored.

Because prolonged bed rest can result in a loss of physical fitness and other health problems, a person who does not have any complications from a heart attack is usually allowed to get up and sit in a chair and begin passive exercises. Physical activity is gradually increased, and the person may leave the hospital when he or she is able to walk without assistance. The doctor will probably prescribe a cardiac risk-reduction and rehabilitation program. The program will probably consist of diet modification, exercise, and a weight-loss plan if the person is overweight. Losing weight helps to reduce the heart's workload. If heart function returns to normal, the person can usually resume his or her previous activity level within 6 weeks of the heart attack. He or she can resume sexual activity at this time.

Depending on the person's condition, the doctor may recommend regular exercise such as walking or bicycling. If necessary, the doctor may prescribe medication to maintain adequate heart function and control high blood pressure. The person may have to reduce or eliminate alcohol consumption. Also, if the person smokes, the doctor will advise him or her to quit smoking immediately. The doctor may recommend a smoking-cessation product such as nicotine gum, a nicotine patch, or medication, or smoking-cessation classes if the person has difficulty quitting on his or her own. The doctor will also prescribe regular office visits, including periodic stress tests.

The doctor may recommend stress reduction and relaxation techniques if the person's previous lifestyle was stressful or if he or she has problems dealing with stress. A person who has survived a heart attack will have lingering concerns about his or her future health and survival. Some people may become depressed because they feel weak and vulnerable, especially if the heart attack leads to lifestyle changes, a job change, or even a job loss. As the caregiver, you should empathize with the person, but you must resist the urge to become overprotective. Offer support, encouragement, and a positive attitude to help promote the person's recovery. Psychological counseling may be necessary if the person resists making necessary lifestyle changes, or if fear of another possible heart attack interferes with his or her ability to function and resume a normal life. If this is the case, or if your loved one is depressed, ask your doctor for a referral to a mental health professional.

Stroke

Stroke is the sudden interruption of blood flow to a part of the brain, usually causing problems with sensation, movement, and function in areas of the body controlled by that part of the brain. Stroke can result from diseases and conditions such as hypertension (high blood pressure), diabetes, cardiac arrhythmia (abnormal heart rate or rhythm), and atherosclerosis (formation of fatty deposits called plaques in the artery walls, which interferes with normal blood flow). A transient ischemic attack (TIA) is a mild form of stroke in which temporary interruption of blood flow can cause temporary impairment of vision, speech, sensation, or movement.

People who have strokes often need physical therapy,

occupational therapy, or speech therapy, or a combination of these, to complete their recovery. These therapies may be performed in the hospital, at a rehabilitation facility, or at a skilled nursing facility that offers these services. After leaving the healthcare facility, the person may need to continue rehabilitation at home. A visiting nurse association can provide these services, or, in some cases, the caregiver may be taught to provide the home therapy.

The therapist or caregiver will help the person perform the program of exercises that has been designed specifically to maintain or improve his or her current level of functioning. Consistency and follow-through are very important for the exercises to be effective. The therapy program should also include helping the person relearn lost or impaired skills, such as performing activities of daily living (including bathing, grooming, and dressing). Do not be discouraged if the person initially has difficulty walking or talking normally. Therapy, which requires time and patience, is the key to regaining these essential skills.

Although it may seem easier and quicker to do everything for the person, doing so will make him or her dependent on you and can interfere with or prevent his or her recovery. Allow adequate time to help the person bathe and dress in the morning to ensure that he or she can accomplish these activities with a minimum of stress and anxiety. Let the person perform as many tasks as possible instead of doing them yourself and rushing through them to save time. A relaxed, caring, and instructive atmosphere will enable a person who has had a stroke to maintain dignity and self-esteem while taking positive steps toward recovery and regaining as much independence as possible. The person may be angry about having had a stroke or depressed about his or her rate of recovery. If symptoms of depression (see page 23) continue for weeks, talk to the doctor.

Reestablishing a Toilet Routine after a Stroke

After a stroke, it may take some time to reestablish a toilet routine. During the day, help the person onto the toilet or commode every 2 hours. Have him or her drink plenty of fluids (at least eight glasses daily, 8 ounces each) to produce enough urine to fill the bladder, stimulate receptors in the brain, and signal the urge to urinate. Recognizing the sensation of a full bladder will, over time, enable the person to control urination.

Reestablishing a toilet routine also requires the person to sit on the toilet or commode at regular intervals to have a bowel movement. Note the person's usual time or times for moving his or her bowels each day and help him or her onto the toilet around these times to establish a routine. If the person is able to communicate the need to have a bowel movement, this should be relatively easy. However, if the person is unable to speak or understand speech because of the stroke, you may need to work out a different communication system, such as writing things down. During the course of reestablishing a toilet routine, the person may need to wear absorbent disposable briefs. Using nonprescription stool softeners after a stroke can often help prevent straining during a bowel movement.

Seizures

Seizures are caused by uncontrolled electrical activity in the brain that can result in temporary loss of consciousness and involuntary muscle contractions. Some people who have had strokes have seizures. Be prepared to deal with seizures if they occur.

Some seizures are characterized by purposeless behavior such as wandering and mental confusion. Seizures can be partial or generalized, and some people experience more than one type of seizure. Partial seizures can result in stiffening or jerking of an arm or leg, usually accompanied by a tingling feeling in the same area. Generalized seizures affect a larger area, sometimes the entire body.

Grand mal seizures are generalized seizures that are often preceded by a recognizable warning, or aura, which can be a sensory perception such as a distinct sound, smell, or visual image. The person falls to the ground, his or her body stiffens, and the muscles contract and relax. Tongue biting, loss of bladder control, labored breathing, and, occasionally, cessation of breathing are characteristics of a grand mal seizure. When the person regains consciousness after about 3 to 5 minutes, he or she may be confused and drowsy. Many people fall asleep after having a grand mal seizure.

Seizures are usually treated with antiseizure medication. A doctor must closely monitor a person who is taking this type of medication. The most important aspect of seizure control is to carefully follow the medication schedule. Making a note of all seizures will help the doctor to adjust dosages or change the medication to control symptoms and the occurrence of seizures. Adverse effects of antiseizure medication include lethargy, difficulty walking, dizziness, uncontrolled eye movements, irritability, nausea, and vomiting. In severe cases, when treatment with antiseizure medication is not effective in eliminating the seizures, surgery may be recommended to remove the portion of the brain that triggers the seizures.

Witnessing a family member or friend having a seizure can be a frightening experience. If a seizure occurs while you are present, stay focused and try not to panic. The most important thing for you to do is to take steps to ensure that the person is safe and is not injured. If the person falls to the floor, try to clear the area of furniture and other obstacles so that he or she will not bump into anything. Loosen tight clothing, especially around the neck, and try to turn the person on his or her side to avoid breathing in vomit. If you or a family member has a seizure for the first time, see a doctor as soon as possible to get a diagnosis.

WARNING: When a person is having a seizure, never attempt to put a spoon or any other object between his or her teeth to force his or her mouth open; the person may bite down on it and be seriously injured.

Status epilepticus is a state of continuous seizure or repeated seizures with no return to consciousness in between. This can occur with all types of seizures. Status epilepticus is a medical emergency that requires immediate treatment. Call 911 or your local emergency medical number immediately.

4

Choosing a
Home Healthcare Provider

Home healthcare agencies provide and coordinate a wide variety of services for people who need care in their home. Ideally, a person's doctor works with the agency to develop an individualized care plan that identifies the types of home care services that are required, the frequency of service, and who will provide the services. The doctor oversees the care plan and reviews it at regular intervals along with personnel from the healthcare agency. The care plan is adjusted to the person's needs and condition. Medicare has set specific guidelines for home healthcare agencies for reviewing care plans for Medicare recipients.

In general, home healthcare agencies provide services that range from semiskilled nursing care to complex therapies and medical treatments, depending on a person's needs. For example, home healthcare agency personnel can make home visits to give medications or to change dressings, or they can teach family members how to provide such care. The agency may also provide more complex treatments, such as intravenous therapy and wound care, and coordinate a complete program of home care, including dental care, vision care, foot care, and rehabilitation services. In many communities, home healthcare agencies provide physical therapy, speech therapy, occupational therapy, respiratory therapy, counseling, social services, and nutrition programs. Some agencies provide home health aides to help with daily tasks and household chores.

In some cases, Medicare, Medicaid, or private health insurance may pay for all or a portion of these services. Check in advance with the person's insurer to determine if costs for these services are covered. To be eligible for Medicare or Medicaid payments, home health agencies are required to meet standards of care that are set by the federal government and are subject to government supervision and regulation. Under Medicare guidelines, a person who receives home healthcare services must be homebound (unable to leave home without the assistance of another person) and may not visit anyone outside the home except for his or her physician. Another Medicare rule states that the person must receive skilled nursing services in the home. This includes care, instruction, and monitoring by a registered nurse, or an exercise program developed by a physical therapist under the direction of a doctor.

Most of the services described here are available in some form in most cities and many larger towns in the United States. For a referral, talk to your doctor or hospital social worker or discharge planner. For a list of licensed agencies or for additional information, contact your local Area Agency on Aging, or your city, county, or state department of public health or department of social services.

Home healthcare associations as well as hospice associations in your state have current listings of licensed agencies and can recommend an agency that provides the services you need.

Home healthcare agencies are also listed in your local yellow pages under headings such as "home care," "home health services," "hospice," and "nurses."

Home healthcare agencies are divided into the following general categories:

- **Proprietary agencies** are for-profit organizations that can bill Medicare for their visits. However, federal regulations do not permit these agencies to make a profit on the Medicare portion of the business.

- **Facility-based agencies** are part of a larger organization such as a nursing home, hospital, rehabilitation center, or health maintenance organization (HMO).

- **Government agencies** are organizations that are managed by state, county, or local health departments.

- **Visiting nurse associations** are usually nonprofit community-based organizations operated by a governing board made up of healthcare professionals and members of the local community. These organizations often receive financial assistance from the United Way.

- **Private, nonprofit home healthcare agencies** are organizations owned and operated by an individual or a group of people and are usually independent. They are typically funded by the federal government or by religious organizations.

Finding a home healthcare provider that is right for your loved one requires some research. No matter what type of care your loved one needs, ask the following basic questions before selecting a home healthcare provider:

- Is the provider licensed and registered with the appropriate regulatory agencies in your state?

- Is the provider accredited by an appropriate agency? Accrediting agencies include the Accreditation Commission for Home Care, Inc.; the Community Health Accreditation Program; the Joint Commission on Accreditation of Healthcare Organizations; the National Committee for Quality Assurance; and the National HomeCaring Council Division of the Foundation for Hospice and Homecare.

- How long has the provider been in operation?

- What is the provider's reputation in the community? Ask your doctor if he or she has an opinion about this provider.

- What services are offered?

- What are the fees for the services you require? Will your health insurance cover these fees? What are the billing procedures?

- Is the provider Medicare-certified?

- Does the provider carefully screen potential staff members?

- What types of training do staff members receive? Are skills updated on a regular basis?

- Does the provider regularly evaluate staff performance? What is the rate of staff turnover?

- Do staff members work closely with the doctor and family members to develop an ongoing care plan?

- Does the agency provide required equipment?

- Do staff members train family members to perform caregiving duties?

- Are staff members available on weekends and holidays?

- How does the provider handle emergencies? Does it have a 24-hour phone number for emergency assistance?

- How does the provider handle questions and complaints from customers? How are problems resolved?

- What is the provider's refund policy? As an example, if you pay for a month and your family member changes agencies, what adjustment will be made?

Request a list of references from each potential provider. Contacting everyone on these lists for information will help you form an overall impression of the provider. Ask references about the quality of the services they received and about the provider's reliability. The more thorough your research, the more likely you will be able to locate and choose an appropriate, high-quality home healthcare provider that you and your loved one will be happy with.

Visiting Nurse Associations

Visiting nurse associations are the most frequently used home healthcare agencies. In fact, the terms "home healthcare agency" and "visiting nurse association" are often used interchangeably. A visiting nurse association is an organization of registered nurses and other health professionals who specialize in providing intermittent individual home healthcare. Registered nurses (RNs) and licensed practical nurses (LPNs) provide skilled nursing care such as intravenous therapy, nutritional therapy (tube feeding), wound care, and injections. An LPN provides care under the supervision of a registered nurse.

Anyone—a caregiver, family member, or friend—can initiate contact with a visiting nurse association to request its services; the agency will then contact the person's physician for further instructions. The agency supervises and monitors its personnel and coordinates and provides care under the direction of the person's physician. Most visiting nurse associations provide other services in addition to skilled nursing care in the home. These services may include mental health nursing, physical therapy, occupational therapy, speech therapy, respiratory therapy, social services, dietary assistance, and homemaker services.

Third-party payers such as Medicare, Medicaid, HMOs, and private insurance companies usually cover the costs of services provided by a visiting nurse association, as long as these services are prescribed by a doctor and the person meets specific eligibility requirements. The person and his or her family may choose to pay out-of-pocket expenses for home healthcare services that are not covered by a third-party payer. In some cases, state or local government agencies or community organizations may provide or pay for necessary care that is not covered by third-party payers.

Visiting nurse associations provide home healthcare that enables a person to remain at home and receive needed treatment, monitoring, and supervision. These services do not replace visits to the doctor's office, but they are an important supplement to such visits. The nurse will visit the person's home according to a schedule determined by the nurse and the person's physician. If problems occur between visits, the person or his or her caregivers must notify the nurse or the doctor. Most visiting nurse associations have an answering service and a nurse on call to handle urgent matters that arise before or after regular working hours. During home visits, the nurse will provide instructions about when and whom to call if any problems arise. He or she will inform the physician about the person's condition and will alert the doctor about any significant change. The doctor may then alter the care plan by, for example, changing medications or adjusting the dosage to meet the person's changing needs.

Many visiting nurse associations now provide complex, high-tech treatments such as intravenous medications, fluid replacement, hyperalimentation (providing nutrients to a person who is undernourished or who cannot eat), and blood transfusions in a person's home. Home healthcare usually is discontinued when the person's condition has stabilized, when the course of treatment is finished, or when the person has reached his or her maximum level of function.

Visiting nurse associations also provide the assistance of home health aides, who work under the supervision of a registered nurse. Home health aides can help the person sit up in bed, get in and out of bed, walk, eat, and use a toilet, commode, or bedpan. They can also perform personal care tasks such as bathing, dressing, and grooming. The nurse gives the home health aide a list of tasks to perform and monitors the aide's performance at least once every 14 days. The nurse is responsible for making any necessary changes in the aide's duties.

A person who is receiving care from a home healthcare provider has the right to expect respectful, conscientious service administered consistently by the same small group of people over time. It facilitates good continuity of care when the nurses become familiar with the person and his or her condition and care plan. If a different nurse visits each time, contact the agency and request the same nurse for each visit. If this is not possible, consider switching to another agency. Ideally, a trusting relationship should develop between the person being cared for and his or her nurse and caregivers. In addition, the agency should return all of your telephone calls and answer all of your questions satisfactorily.

If you are ever dissatisfied for any reason with the performance of a home healthcare provider, discuss your concerns with the nurse, the nursing supervisor, or your doctor. You should expect paid caregivers who work for home healthcare agencies to adhere to the following basic rules:

- Arrive on time for work.
- Do not sleep on the job.

- Do not smoke in the home.
- Do not borrow money from a client.
- Do not make personal phone calls, or limit the number of calls and the length of each one (as agreed on).
- Do not borrow a car or other vehicle from a client.

Protecting Your Loved One

Although most people have a trusting relationship with their home healthcare providers, it is always a good idea to take precautions to minimize problems. To reduce the risk of theft, limit the access of home healthcare providers to specific areas of the house or apartment. Take an inventory of your loved one's property and check it on a regular basis. Never leave valuables such as cash, jewelry, credit cards, checkbooks, or collectibles lying about. Keep them in a secure place, such as a home safe or a safety deposit box in a bank. Also, carefully monitor all household expenses to keep track of any unexpected costs, such as an unusually high telephone bill.

Do not allow a home healthcare provider to have access to your loved one's money or bank accounts. If the caregiver needs to make purchases such as food or medication, give him or her enough money to cover those expenses and request receipts for all purchases. All checks made out to your loved one should be deposited directly into his or her bank account. You should deposit them personally, rather than delegating this task to a home health aide.

To help ensure your loved one's safety and security, make sure that you know exactly who is in the home at all times. Under no circumstances should professional caregivers be allowed to bring other people into the home. If your loved one lives alone, make unannounced visits and phone calls so you can monitor the situation.

Home health agencies are liable for the care they provide. If you want to file an official complaint, contact one or more of the following:

- The agency's top administrator
- Your state or local licensing or regulating agency for home healthcare providers
- Your state or local Medicare hot line
- Your state or local department of public health
- Your local Better Business Bureau

In addition, many states provide a hot line you can call to report dissatisfaction with home healthcare services. Check your telephone book or call directory assistance for that number and the numbers of the agencies listed above. All serious complaints should be promptly investigated by the appropriate licensing and regulating agency in your state.

Social Service Agencies

Social service agencies are organizations that deal with the social, emotional, and environmental problems associated with illness, disability, and aging. Social workers are trained to provide guidance, support, counseling, and hands-on assistance to people in a wide variety of circumstances. Social workers can assess individual needs and make arrangements or referrals for needed services, such as transportation and financial assistance. Some social service agencies specialize in a particular service, such as finding new housing for older people and relocating them. Others may provide trained companions to call or visit older people who are homebound, or provide legal assistance and advice. Charges for these services often are determined by a sliding scale based on the person's ability to pay. Some services may be provided free of charge. Social service agencies are listed in your telephone book. Hospital social service departments provide these services for their patients.

Medication and Infusion Therapy Services

Medication and infusion therapy services provide medication and equipment for people who are receiving intravenous drug therapy or nutritional therapy (tube feeding) at home. Staff nurses come to a person's home to set up the equipment and teach the person and his or her caregivers how to administer these therapies. In most cases, Medicaid and private insurance cover the cost of medication and infusion therapy services. Medicare covers the costs of nutritional therapy and some intravenous drug therapies based on strict eligibility guidelines.

Community and Volunteer Organizations

Community and volunteer organizations such as churches or synagogues or local service clubs may be able to assist you. Various public and private organizations may provide a variety of specialized home-care services, some of which may be offered free of charge. For example, volunteer visitors and companions from these organizations come to a homebound person's home on a regular basis to spend some time and check on his or her status. Ask your doctor or social worker for recommendations.

Volunteer health organizations, such as the American Cancer Society and the Easter Seal Society, often have programs that benefit people who are ill or disabled. They may be able to lend you equipment and provide you with helpful information. Check the white pages of your telephone book.

Homemaker and Home Repair Services

Homemaker services are private or nonprofit fee-for-service organizations that provide the services of trained homemakers or housekeepers. These workers perform chores that may include general housecleaning, preparing meals, doing laundry, shopping, and performing yard work—tasks generally geared to maintaining the home. Before service begins, make a list of all the tasks that you would like the homemaker to perform. This will ensure that all your needs are met and avoid misunderstandings about the arrangement.

Make sure that the organization providing homemaker services is licensed and bonded. This will ensure, for example, that the agency will reimburse you for missing or broken items. Some agencies perform criminal background checks on their potential employees; make sure that the agency you choose performs this important screening. Ask to interview several prospective employees before selecting an agency. You are free to change your mind if the employee you choose does not meet your standards for any reason.

In general, the person or his or her family must pay out-of-pocket costs for homemaker services. Some private insurance policies may cover part or all of the costs of these services. In some cases, state or local government agencies or community organizations may provide or pay for homemaker services.

Home maintenance and repair services are available in many communities. Workers may perform tasks such as installing smoke detectors, washing windows, cleaning gutters, and painting. These services are often provided by community or volunteer organizations and are often free of charge. Call your local government office and ask if any of these services are available in your community.

Special Meal Services

Meal services such as Meals on Wheels provide home delivery of nutritionally balanced hot and cold meals for older and disabled people who are not able to prepare their own meals. Fees for this service are often based on a person's ability to pay. Because the demand for such services is high in some communities, preference may be given to people with limited income.

In other communities, anyone who can pay the full fee is eligible. Special diets require a written order from a doctor.

In some communities, senior citizen centers offer lunch and dinner in a group setting. Meals are often free or available for a small charge based on a person's ability to pay. Older people who are able to travel to such centers get a balanced meal and also have the opportunity to socialize with others. In some cases, transportation to the center may be available. Ask your doctor or social worker about special meal services in your community.

Transportation Services

Transportation services for older or disabled people are provided at reasonable cost in many communities. This is useful for people who cannot drive or use regular public transportation, or who depend on friends, relatives, or neighbors for rides. Possible modes of transportation are taxi, van, ambulance, and Medicar. A Medicar is a van that transports people in wheelchairs to their doctor's office and back home. Cost includes pickup and mileage fees. This service is useful for people who cannot get into a taxi or a car. Medicaid sometimes pays for Medicar service.

Ambulance service is appropriate for people who are unable to use a taxi, car, or Medicar. These people might require an ambulance to travel to and from the hospital and to go to their physician's office. Medicare may pay for transportation to and from the hospital but will not cover the cost of an ambulance to the doctor's office; this expense must be paid out of pocket. Medicar and ambulance services are listed in your telephone book.

Medicaid usually covers the cost of taxi service for people who cannot get to their doctor's office on public transportation. Those who are able to get to the doctor's office on public transportation but choose to use taxi service instead must pay for the taxi service out of pocket. Many communities provide transportation for disabled or physically challenged people through either public or private agencies. Volunteer transportation services are available in some areas. Some medical facilities and clinics that treat older people provide transportation, either free or at a nominal cost. Ask your doctor or social worker about transportation services that may be available in your community.

Adult Day Care Programs

Adult day care programs are designed primarily for older people who need some limited supervision but are able to care for themselves and want to remain at home instead of living in a nursing home. These programs may provide physician-directed medical and rehabilitative services or supervised recreational and social activities. Adult day care programs are often used to provide respite for caregivers. Day care may be available from 1 to 5 days per week, depending on the program. Some community organizations, senior citizen centers, or church-related groups provide this service. The cost of adult day care varies nationwide. Some adult day care programs do not charge any fees for the services they provide. When fees are charged, they often are determined on a sliding scale, based on a person's ability to pay. In some states, Medicaid covers the cost of adult day care for people who meet specific eligibility requirements. Ask your doctor to recommend an adult day care program in your area.

Friends and Relatives

Friends and relatives can be a great resource when caring for someone at home. Make a list of all the tasks that need to be done—such as errands, telephone calls, meals, chores, and social visits and transportation—and, when people ask what they can do to help, offer them a choice. Update the list as needed. With a list at hand, you are more likely to be in a position to take advantage of offers of assistance. Because friends and relatives are concerned and eager to help in any way they can, don't feel that you are imposing on them.

Drugstores and Medical Supply Companies

Drugstores and medical supply companies carry a wide selection of home care equipment and supplies, such as hospital beds, wheelchairs, walkers, ventilators, catheters, commodes, bedpans, and handheld urinals. These providers usually deliver and set up the equipment in the home and show the person and his or her caregivers how to use it properly. You may want to consider renting, rather than buying, the equipment you need, especially if you need it only temporarily. Also, renting gives you the opportunity to test various types of equipment before deciding on what to buy. Medicare, Medicaid, and private insurance plans usually cover the cost of home-care equipment and medical supplies when these items are medically necessary and have been prescribed by a doctor.

Hospice

Hospice refers to services that are designed to meet the special needs of people who are terminally ill. Hospice care focuses on the relief of symptoms. The goal is to allow a dying person to spend his or her last days as comfortably as possible with family and friends in a secure, caring environment. These services may be provided at home, in a nursing home, or, in some cases, for a few days in the hospital. A doctor's authorization is required to place a person in a hospice program; in most cases, a person is eligible for hospice when a doctor has determined that he or she is not expected to live longer than 6 months.

Various types of hospice programs offer various types of care—from basic emotional support to complex medical services. Most hospice programs are Medicare certified and are licensed and regulated by the state in which they operate. Regardless of the level of care provided, trained professionals work closely with the dying person and his or her loved ones and are available to assist the family 24 hours a day. Some hospice programs may also provide grief counseling for family members after their loved one has died.

Medicare covers the full cost of Medicare-certified hospice care. Medicaid programs in many states, most private health insurance plans, and some HMOs and other managed care plans also cover the cost of hospice care. The person or his or her family may pay out-of-pocket expenses for hospice care if the person is not eligible for Medicare or Medicaid hospice benefits, or if his or her private insurance or managed care plan does not cover the cost. Because most hospice programs provide care based on need rather than on a person's ability to pay, cost is determined on a sliding scale. In some cases, hospice care may be available free of charge to people who have limited resources. Find out about a particular hospice program's payment policies in advance.

5

Paying for Home Healthcare

Home healthcare can be expensive, with costs varying according to the level of care provided and the length of time it is needed. Various public and private insurers, programs, and organizations may cover all or part of the costs of home healthcare. Because eligibility requirements and the coverage of services and costs vary from one payer to another, it is very important for caregivers to become familiar with their loved one's insurance plan or plans.

Potential third-party payers include Medicare, Medicaid, state-funded healthcare, private insurance plans (including Medicare supplemental insurance and long-term care insurance), the Department of Veterans Affairs, Workers' Compensation, CHAMPUS (Civilian Health and Medical Program of the Uniformed Services), managed care plans, and various community and volunteer organizations. In general, home health agencies bill Medicare and Medicaid directly for services that are covered by those programs. You can also arrange to have these agencies bill other third-party payers directly. Costs that are not covered by Medicare, Medicaid, or another third-party payer are usually billed directly to the client, who must pay them out of pocket.

Medicare

The Health Insurance for the Aged and Disabled Act (commonly called the Medicare Act) has made a broad program of healthcare available to nearly every American age 65 and older. The program also covers people under 65 who have a disability or end-stage kidney disease. Medicare is divided into Part A and Part B. Medicare Part A is financed through payroll contributions paid by employees, employers, and people who are self-employed. Part A covers hospital costs. Medicare Part B is financed by monthly premiums paid by people who voluntarily enroll, and by the federal government, which contributes a portion from general revenues. Part B covers physician costs.

Medicare has strict eligibility guidelines. The cost of home healthcare for people age 65 and over is usually covered by Medicare Part A when the services are provided intermittently or part-time, are prescribed by a doctor, and are provided by a Medicare-certified agency. For continued coverage, the doctor must also follow federal guidelines and review the person's care plan at regular intervals. Medicare may cover the cost of services such as skilled nursing care, rehabilitation therapies, and medical supplies and equipment. Hospice care is covered by Medicare Part A when a physician certifies that a person is terminally ill and has 6 months or less to live. If necessary, this certification can be renewed every 6 months for continued Medicare coverage. To receive the Medicare Hospice Benefit, the person must sign a statement forfeiting his or her rights to other Medicare benefits for people who are terminally ill.

For information about Medicare eligibility and benefits, call the Social Security Administration at (800) 772-1213, or contact the Health Care Financing Administration at (800) MEDICARE (633-4227).

Medicare Supplemental Insurance

For Medicare beneficiaries, Medicare supplemental insurance policies (sometimes called Medigap insurance) may pay for some home healthcare services that are not covered by Medicare. To be eligible for Medicare supplemental insurance coverage, a person's doctor must prescribe these services in combination with other services that are covered by Medicare. These policies are designed to cover the costs of short-term care, such as recovery from injury, major surgery, or acute illness. They do not cover the costs of long-term care.

Medicaid

Medicaid is a state program that provides health insurance for low-income residents. Both the federal and state governments provide financing for the Medicaid program. Eligibility requirements vary from state to state, but people who qualify are generally those who already receive federal assistance payments such as Aid to Families with Dependent Children (AFDC) and Social Security income. Others who may receive Medicaid home healthcare benefits include people who are disabled, older people whose incomes fall below federal poverty levels but are too high to qualify for federal assistance payments, and people under age 21 whose incomes qualify them for AFDC but who are not eligible for AFDC for other reasons.

According to federal Medicaid guidelines, covered services

include part-time skilled nursing care, home health aides, medications, and medical equipment and supplies. Some states also cover the cost of medical social services, hearing care, and rehabilitation therapies. Check with your local Medicaid office to find out which services are covered in your state.

If a person receives both Medicare and Medicaid benefits, then Medicare takes precedence, and the healthcare agency will bill any charges to the Medicare program first. A Medicaid hospice benefit is available in most states, and it covers the cost of the same services as the Medicare hospice benefit.

Department of Veterans Affairs

The Department of Veterans Affairs (VA; formerly known as the Veterans Administration) covers the cost of home healthcare for eligible veterans who are at least 50 percent disabled, if the disability is service-related. To be covered, home care must be authorized by a doctor and provided through a VA hospital. Contact the nearest Department of Veterans Affairs Regional Office for additional information about benefits and eligibility.

Long-term Care Insurance

Long-term care insurance was originally designed to cover the costs of catastrophic care, such as a long stay in a nursing facility. Today, some long-term care insurance policies also provide coverage for certain home healthcare services. Long-term care insurance is usually available only to people who are in generally good health at the time they purchase the policy. Coverage varies considerably from one policy to another. The premiums are high, especially if you purchase the policy after age 60, and like any insurance policy, you must study the plan carefully to be sure you understand what is covered and what the limitations

are. You will find big differences in the dollar benefits, in defi-
nitions of covered facilities, in the length of time benefits are
paid, and in eligibility for benefits. Check your policy or talk to
your insurer to determine the extent of your benefits.

Workers' Compensation

Workers' Compensation may cover the cost of home-care services that are needed as a result of a work-related injury or illness. Workers' Compensation also covers the cost of
rehabilitation. To be eligible for home care or rehabilitation
benefits, the person first must prove that he or she is injured or
ill, that the injury or illness is work-related, and that this has
resulted in medical or rehabilitation expenses. If your loved one
has a work-related injury or illness, contact his or her
employer's personnel office or human resources department for
information on eligibility for benefits and how to file a claim.

CHAMPUS

CHAMPUS (Civilian Health and Medical Program of the Uniformed Services) covers all or part of the cost of some home
healthcare services for dependents of active military personnel
and retired military personnel and their dependents or survivors. The Uniformed Services includes the Army, Navy, Air
Force, Marines, Coast Guard, National Oceanic and Atmos-
pheric Administration, and Public Health Service. CHAMPUS
also covers the costs of hospice care. To submit a claim, the person must be enrolled in the Defense Enrollment Eligibility
Reporting System (DEERS). Contact any local military personnel office for additional information about eligibility and
benefits.

Community and Volunteer Organizations

Community organizations, such as religious institutions and local service clubs (such as Rotary, Elks, and Kiwanis), and local chapters of national volunteer health organizations (such as the American Cancer Society, the Easter Seal Society, and the Alzheimer's Association) may provide financial assistance for home healthcare services for eligible people. For more information about financial assistance available from these organizations, contact them directly (check your local telephone book) or ask your doctor, visiting nurse, or hospital social worker for a recommendation. Other good sources of information about these groups include your local Area Agency on Aging (see page 108) and the local chapter of the United Way (check your local telephone book).

6

Rehabilitation Services

Rehabilitation services include physical, occupational, speech, respiratory, and vocational therapies. A person who has been disabled by disease, injury, or stroke, or who has had certain types of surgery such as hip replacement is likely to need one or more of these therapies to promote recovery. Rehabilitation begins at the hospital, and the person continues the therapy at home. Caregivers are encouraged to play an active role in the rehabilitation process and are usually trained to perform or assist with certain treatments.

Health insurance coverage is an important consideration for a person who needs rehabilitation. Many insurance plans limit the types of treatments (including rehabilitation therapies) and the number of visits or sessions they cover. Some plans may also require policyholders to use designated facilities or service providers. Certification, which indicates that a therapy program meets certain standards or follows specific guidelines, may also be a requirement for insurance coverage, as is the case for Medicare. Even if the insurer does not require certification, it is a good idea to determine in advance if the therapist you have selected has appropriate training and supervision. Check with your loved one's physician or visiting nurse for recommendations.

Whichever type of therapy your loved one needs, get involved with it yourself. Ask each therapist to recommend ways in which you can support and reinforce the progress and goals of treatment. For example, you may be able to assist with performing specific exercises on days when the therapist does not visit. You can also play an important role as "cheerleader," providing motivation and encouragement even when progress is slow or limited. Everyone involved in the person's care can help by maintaining a positive, supportive attitude.

Also consider ways in which you can make the most efficient use of a therapist's presence. For example, if you do not have to assist during a therapy session, you may be able to use this time to relax or to complete an important chore or errand. Some possibilities for relaxation include reading, taking a walk, talking with a friend, or gardening. Both you and your loved one will benefit when you make good use of these opportunities to take a break.

Remember that working with a therapist, while often rewarding, can also be difficult. Hard work or slow progress can be tiring and frustrating and may draw attention away from the goals of the therapy, causing your loved one to focus instead on his or her illness, injury, or disability. It is important for all participants to understand, from the outset, the realistic goals of the therapy and what it will take to reach those goals. It is also important to acknowledge the potential for setbacks during the recovery process so that your loved one will not give up if a setback occurs. It must also be made clear that, for some people, recovery may be limited. To help ensure the success of any therapy, it is crucial to keep the lines of communication open and to always be willing to discuss your loved one's feelings and concerns as he or she works toward recovery.

Physical Therapy

Physical therapy can help a person regain physical strength and mobility. The goal of physical therapy is to restore normal function after illness or injury. For example, a person who is recovering from hip replacement surgery will need to perform specific exercises to rebuild the muscles and regain flexibility in the hip area. He or she will also need to learn new ways to sit, walk, climb stairs, and perform other daily activities, such as getting in and out of a car. A person with more limited physical abilities may have simpler but still important needs, such as learning how to sit up in a chair or maneuver safely from a bed to a commode.

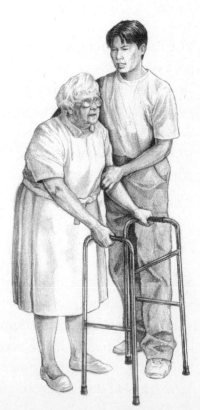

A physical therapist is a trained professional who provides treatment such as exercise, massage, manipulation, heat, cold, water, and electrical current. A physical therapist can also help a person learn to use a prosthesis such as an artificial arm or leg, or a cane, crutches, or a walker (see illustration). Some physical therapists have been certified as geriatric specialists by the American Physical Therapy Association to work primarily with older people.

Occupational Therapy

Occupational therapy is provided by trained professionals who help people who have been disabled by injury or illness regain muscle control and coordination, perform everyday tasks, and, if possible, return to work. An occupational therapist can help people adjust to and compensate for injuries that may have affected their ability to feed, dress, or bathe themselves. Treatment often begins in the hospital and may continue at an outpatient clinic or in the person's home.

Vocational Therapy

Vocational therapy can help a person relearn skills that were part of his or her former job, learn new job skills, and identify new employment opportunities. A vocational therapist can provide guidance, training, and employment placement assistance. The goal of such programs is to enable people to function as well as possible within the limits of their capabilities. A person who has had a serious head injury, a spinal injury, or a stroke may benefit from this type of therapy.

Speech Therapy

Speech therapy helps people regain speech skills and their ability to communicate effectively following a disease or trauma such as a stroke, brain tumor, or head injury. Speech therapists are also trained to assist people who are having problems with breathing, swallowing, and muscle control (as it relates to specific parts of the mouth and throat). The therapist works closely with caregivers, family, and friends to encourage them to actively participate in the person's treatment and recovery.

Respiratory Therapy

Respiratory therapy provides care for people who have breathing problems, including people who have respiratory diseases such as asthma or emphysema, who are recovering from major surgery, or who must breathe with the assistance of a ventilator (a device that pumps air into the lungs). Respiratory therapists provide oxygen, medication, and moisture to the lungs. They also are trained to help loosen and drain sputum and other secretions from clogged lungs.

7

Caring for an Older Person Who Lives Alone

Older people want to remain independent for as long as possible. Factors that can interfere with an older person's continued independence include physical or mental changes with age, the safety of the home environment, and medical problems that affect his or her ability to function on his or her own.

Modifying the Home Environment

A safe environment is often the most immediate concern when an older person lives alone. Take a careful look around your loved one's house or apartment building and neighborhood. What are the neighbors like? Is there much crime in the area? If necessary, you may want to consider relocating your loved one, or modifying the home to make it a safer place. These recommendations also apply to your own home if an older person lives with you. Carefully and thoroughly inspect the house or apartment, and take the following steps to ensure your loved one's safety:

- Modify the home as needed to help prevent falls (see below).
- Install smoke alarms, especially near bedrooms and the kitchen, and a carbon monoxide detector on each floor. Check the batteries frequently and replace them on the same day every year whether they need it or not.
- Plan an escape route in case of fire, and have regular fire drills.
- Keep a clear path to all doors that lead outside.
- Set the temperature of the water heater below 110 degrees Fahrenheit.
- Keep a fire extinguisher in the kitchen and learn how to use and maintain it properly.
- Repair or replace any electrical appliances that have frayed wires or damaged plugs.
- Check for overloaded electrical outlets.
- Remove electrical cords from underneath rugs or carpets.
- Install dead-bolt locks on outside doors and sturdy locks on all windows.
- Have the furnace and thermostat inspected regularly by a qualified, reliable heating professional.

Preventing Falls

For an older person, even a minor fall can cause serious injury. Many older people develop a fear of falling and become increasingly less active. Inactivity can actually increase a person's risk of falling and can lead to serious health problems, such as deep vein thrombosis (formation of blood clots in deep-lying veins, usually in the legs). Inactivity also can diminish a person's quality of life.

Age-related changes, such as vision problems, muscle weakness, and joint pain caused by arthritis, can increase a person's chances of falling. Some diseases and conditions, such as Parkinson's disease, diabetes, peripheral vascular disease, and heart disease, can also increase the risk. An older person may have problems when walking or using a cane, walker, wheelchair, or braces, which can also increase his or her chances of falling.

Some medications, such as tranquilizers, sedatives, and antipsychotic drugs, can impair a person's alertness and contribute to falls. Antihypertensive medications also present a risk because they can cause abnormally low blood pressure when a person stands or sits up quickly (called postural hypotension). This sudden change in blood pressure can cause dizziness and fainting.

Taking Steps to Prevent Falls

Carefully and thoroughly inspect your loved one's house or apartment and make all necessary changes to help prevent falls. Here are some things you can do:

- Make sure that light switches are located within easy reach of doorways so that the person does not have to cross a dark room to turn on a light. Note that lighting that is too dim or too bright can impair an older person's vision, thereby increasing the risk of falling.

- Be sure that carpets and rugs have slip-resistant backing or that they are tacked down to prevent trips and slips. Remove unnecessary loose rugs, mats, and runners.

- Arrange the furniture so that the person has a clear, unobstructed path from one place to another. Take special care with placement of furniture with sharp or pointed corners and low-rise items such as ottomans and coffee tables, which are easy to bump into or fall over. Remove any furniture that is not being used. Provide a remote control for the television. Keep hallways clear and uncluttered.

- Keep telephone and electrical cords out of pathways.

- Provide sturdy handrails on both sides of all stairways, 30 inches above the steps. Use nonskid treads on all bare steps. If a stairway is carpeted, make sure that the carpeting is tacked down securely on every step. Do not put loose rugs at the top or bottom of stairways. All stairways should be well lit. Make sure there are no toys or other items on the stairs. If the person can no longer climb the stairs, it may be possible to have an electric lift chair installed. Another possible solution is to move the person's bedroom to the first floor, but only if there is a bathroom on that floor.

- Make sure chairs and tables are sturdy, stable, and balanced in case the person leans on them for support.

- Place a lamp within reach of the person's bed and night-lights along the pathways between the bedrooms and the bathroom. Install a night-light in the bathroom.

- Set the thermostat at a warm temperature (at least 72 degrees Fahrenheit) to help keep an older person's joints from stiffening.

- In the bedroom, place guardrails on the bed to help the person get in and out of bed. A sturdy chair placed at the bedside can serve a similar purpose. Place a telephone with volume control and a lighted dial next to the bed.

- In the kitchen, place a nonslip rubber mat on the floor in front of the sink. Clean up spills on the floor and countertops immediately. Keep frequently used items within easy reach to avoid having to bend or climb up on a chair or stepladder to reach them. Be sure that your loved one wears rubber-soled shoes around the house.

- In the bathroom, put a nonslip rubber mat or nonslip adhesive strips on the floor of the tub or shower. Install handrails and grab bars on the walls around the toilet and along the bathtub. Place a nonslip bath mat on the floor by the tub or shower; tile floors can be especially slippery when wet. For some people, a raised toilet seat may be easier to use. Never use towel bars for support; they are not strong enough for this purpose.

- Do not lock the bathroom door. It may be necessary to remove any locks to prevent your loved one from accidentally locking the door.

- Have the doctor review all medications with possible side effects such as drowsiness, dizziness, or fainting to be sure that they are necessary.

- When going outdoors, have the person wear comfortable, sturdy walking shoes with soles that grip the pavement. If he or she uses a cane or walker, make sure that it is sturdy and in good condition. Encourage your loved one to stay indoors, if possible, when the weather is bad, especially when the pavement is wet or icy. During the winter, keep porches, steps, sidewalks, and driveways clear of snow and ice. Always spread sand or salt on icy surfaces.

- An older person who has difficulty walking may benefit from working with a physical therapist, either as an outpatient or through a home healthcare agency. If walking is a problem for your loved one, talk to your doctor about having a gait evaluation and starting an exercise program to improve the person's ability to walk.

In spite of the best preventive measures, falls may still occur. If your loved one falls, keep him or her immobile and try to determine the nature and extent of any injuries. It is important to note that fractures, internal injuries, and head injuries are often not immediately apparent. If you think the person may have a hip, leg, spine, or neck fracture, or any other serious injury, call for emergency medical assistance immediately. Also, any person who has continued pain after a fall should be examined by a doctor as soon as possible.

Personal Emergency Response Systems

Personal emergency response systems (PERS) provide an easy way for an older person to call for help in an emergency. The system includes an electronic monitor (about the size of a small radio or answering machine) that can be placed on a bedside table. The monitor is plugged into an electrical outlet and connected to the person's telephone line. Most systems require the person to push a "help button" to activate the system. There is a button on the monitor and also on a wristband or pendant that the person wears at all times. Some systems may also be voice activated or use motion detectors.

When the system is activated, the signal goes to a monitoring center where a specific set of actions is set into motion. First, the center attempts to contact the person. Depending on the situation (or if the person does not respond), the center either attempts to contact a designated person or series of people (such as a relative, friend, or neighbor) or calls for emergency assistance (from emergency medical services, the fire department, or the police).

Personal emergency response systems are available by subscription in many communities, usually with a one-time installation charge and a monthly fee. In some communities, local hospitals, fire departments, and various community organizations may provide this service. If the person has limited income and assets, the service may be provided for a reduced fee or free of charge. In any case, you should not have to purchase any equipment or sign a long-term contract. Ask your doctor about these systems or contact your local hospital for information.

Providing a Healthy Diet

The ability to prepare or obtain nutritious meals daily plays an important role in determining whether an older person can remain alone in his or her home. If the person can cook but cannot leave the house to shop for food, he or she can phone in an order to a local grocery store for delivery. Groceries can also be ordered on the Internet. Payment can be made by check, cash, or credit or debit card and can usually be paid at the time of delivery. Home-delivered meals such as Meals on Wheels are available at a reasonable cost in many communities. Fees are generally based on a person's ability to pay. The social service department in most hospitals can provide a list of agencies that offer this service.

As we age, our taste buds change and affect the way food tastes. For some people, this can lead to loss of appetite. Other age-related changes include a decrease in the production of saliva, which contributes to difficulty swallowing. When we are older, it may also take longer to digest food. For some people, heartburn or acid reflux (backward flow of stomach contents into the lower part of the esophagus) can cause discomfort or pain after eating. These problems can place an older person at risk for malnutrition and related health problems.

A person may benefit by eating several (five or six) small meals throughout the day instead of three large meals. Have him or her eat plenty of fruits, vegetables, and whole grains, and avoid fried or greasy foods, which can cause bloating and indigestion. Season food with a variety of herbs and spices to enhance its flavor and make everyday meals more appetizing. (Be sure to avoid adding salt or sugar if the person has any dietary restrictions.) Have your loved one sit up for at least 1 hour after finishing a meal to help prevent the discomfort or pain of heartburn or acid reflux.

Calcium Intake for Older People

According to the National Institutes of Health, women who have reached menopause should take in 1,500 milligrams of calcium per day, or 1,000 milligrams per day if they are taking estrogen in hormone replacement therapy. Men age 65 and over should take in 1,500 milligrams of calcium per day. Good sources of calcium include low-fat and nonfat dairy products; green, leafy vegetables; dried peas and beans; and calcium-fortified foods. The chart below shows the approximate amount of calcium in certain foods.

Food	Serving Size	Calcium (in milligrams)
Low-fat or nonfat plain yogurt	1 cup	468
2 percent milk	1 cup	350
Sardines with bones, canned	3 ounces	324
Calcium-fortified orange juice	1 cup	320
1 percent milk or fat-free milk	1 cup	300
Mozzarella cheese, part skim	1 ounce	207
Salmon with bones, canned	3 ounces	181
Tofu (firm)	3 ounces	177
Figs, dried	5 medium	135
Tortilla, corn	2	120
Tortilla, flour	2	106
Great northern beans	½ cup	105
Turnip greens, cooked	½ cup	99
English muffin, plain	1	99
Low-fat cottage cheese	½ cup	69
Orange	1 medium	58
Mustard greens, boiled	½ cup	52
Broccoli, raw	1 cup	42

Our daily calorie needs tend to decrease as we age. For this reason, an older person's diet should be nutritionally dense—that is, small amounts of food should provide large amounts of nutrients. It is also essential for an older person to take in adequate amounts of calcium to facilitate muscle contraction and nerve function, and to help prevent osteoporosis (a condition in which bone becomes thin, brittle, and susceptible to fracture). Older people who have lactose intolerance (an inability to digest dairy products that causes bloating, gas, and diarrhea) may be able to use calcium supplements or commercial products that help with digestion of dairy products. Ask your doctor for advice.

Fluid Intake

To avoid dehydration (abnormally low levels of water in body tissues) and related health problems, it is important to drink an adequate amount of fluid every day. As we age, most people begin to lose the sensation of thirst. Even though body tissues may be in need of water, an older person may not feel thirsty. Therefore, have your loved one drink at regular intervals throughout the day, regardless of whether he or she feels thirsty. Experts recommend that all adults (except for those who are under a doctor's orders to limit their intake of fluids) drink at least eight glasses of fluid, 8 ounces each, every day. Total fluid intake each day can include water, milk, juice, tea, caffeine-free soft drinks, and broth.

If the person you are caring for has memory problems and is likely to forget to drink, leave reminders throughout the house or apartment, including in the kitchen, bathroom, and living room. An easy way to measure daily fluid intake is to fill a 2-quart pitcher with water at the start of each day. Each time the person drinks any type of fluid, pour off the same amount of water from the 2-quart pitcher. If the person has consumed an adequate amount of fluid, the 2-quart pitcher should be empty at the end of the day.

Medications and Older People

Many older people must take several different prescription and nonprescription medications each day. Because these drugs are usually taken according to different schedules, it can be easy for an older person to become confused about which medication to take at what time, or how often to take a given drug. Some people may accidentally skip doses or take extra doses. Some older people may have trouble swallowing their medication. All of these potential problems can present serious health risks. The following tips can help your loved one successfully manage his or her medications:

- Make a list of the medications (both prescription and non-prescription) the person is taking and keep it up-to-date. Tell the doctor about all the drugs your loved one is taking and bring the list (or the containers) along to each office visit. This information helps the doctor prescribe and properly monitor the person's medications.

- If the person has trouble remembering to take medication, try associating doses with specific times of the day, such as getting up in the morning, bedtime, or with meals.

- Keep a medication schedule (in the form of a calendar) and check off each dose as it is taken.

- Use a divided container to prepare the person's doses of medication for the coming week. Containers designed for this purpose are available at drugstores.

- Be sure that the person takes his or her medications exactly as the doctor has prescribed them. Never change the dosage or have the person stop taking any prescribed medication unless the doctor recommends it.

- Ask the doctor to prescribe a medication in the form that is easiest for the person to take. For example, if the person has problems swallowing pills, ask if the medication is available in liquid form.

- If the person has trouble opening containers, ask the pharmacist for containers with easy-open lids rather than child-resistant lids.

- Do not transfer drugs to another container unless you have labeled the container correctly.

- Make sure that the instructions on the labels are easy to read and understand. Do not hesitate to ask the doctor or pharmacist for help.

- Avoid keeping medications on a bedside table. This will keep the person from taking the wrong drug or overdosing when he or she is not fully awake.

- Keep the person's prescriptions up-to-date. If the doctor wants the person to continue taking a medication that is nearing its expiration date, be sure to inform the doctor as soon as possible so that he or she can call the pharmacist to renew the prescription or write a new one.

- Dispose of all unused and expired prescription medications and expired nonprescription medications. Throw them away or flush them down the toilet.

- Be sure that the person never takes any medication that was prescribed for someone else, and never gives his or her medication to anyone else.

Dealing with Constipation

Constipation (infrequent or difficult bowel movements) is a common problem for older people. Possible causes of constipation include age-related changes in the digestive system, decreased activity level, and inadequate daily intake of fluids and dietary fiber. To help prevent constipation, have the person eat plenty of fruits, vegetables, and whole-grain foods every day. Encourage him or her to drink plenty of fluids (at least eight glasses daily, 8 ounces each) and to exercise every day. Include some helpful home remedies—such as prunes or prune juice, applesauce, and bran (in cereal, bread, or muffins)—in your loved one's diet.

Many people mistakenly believe that it is necessary to have a bowel movement every day. Because of this belief, they may take laxatives to ensure that they have a daily bowel movement. But dependence on laxatives can develop quickly and can result in diarrhea, which, in turn, can lead to dehydration. Also, regular use of high-fiber laxatives may result in intestinal obstruction. Stool softeners are sometimes helpful, but they should be taken with an adequate amount of fluid to allow them to work effectively (see package instructions or talk to your doctor or pharmacist). Talk to your doctor if your loved one is having any problems with bowel movements.

Hygiene

An older person who is living alone may have problems with personal hygiene. Bathing and grooming often become difficult as normal, age-related physical changes occur. And familiar activities such as using the bathtub or shower pose serious risks such as falling or being scalded.

Install handrails or grab bars to help prevent bathroom falls. If there are no handrails or grab bars, help the person in and out of the bathtub or shower. Another way to prevent falls is to have the person take a sponge bath while he or she sits on the toilet seat lid or on a bath seat. Different styles of bath seats (with or without backs, with or without padding) designed to meet the person's specific needs are available from drugstores and medical supply companies. If the person cannot bathe and it is difficult for you to assist him or her, consider hiring a home health aide through a home health agency for several hours a few times a week to assist with personal hygiene.

Home Temperature

As we age, our body's ability to regulate temperature can becomes less efficient. Hypothermia (a life-threatening drop in body temperature) can develop quickly in an older person if the temperature of his or her house or apartment is lower than 65 degrees Fahrenheit. Make sure that the heating system in your loved one's home is in proper working order and that there is enough heat throughout the day. This is of particular importance in an apartment building, where tenants usually do not have control over the amount of heat they receive. It is also vital to have the furnace checked on a regular basis for carbon monoxide leaks.

 WARNING: When used improperly, space heaters are a potential cause of burns and fires. If you use a space heater, be sure to keep it at least 3 feet away from anything that might catch fire, such as newspapers, draperies, upholstery, bedding, and walls. Never use an extension cord with an electric space heater. When lighting a gas space heater, strike the match first, then turn on the gas. Never leave a space heater operating when you are not in the room. Also, never use a gas range to heat your home.

Older people are also vulnerable to the effects of a high home temperature, which can lead to life-threatening conditions such as heat exhaustion and heatstroke. Experts strongly recommend that room temperature be maintained at a constant 72 degrees Fahrenheit, if possible. In the summer, fans may be helpful, but in many parts of the United States, air-conditioning may be the only way to keep the temperature at a comfortable level. This can be a serious problem because many older people do not own an air conditioner or cannot afford to pay high electric bills. If this is the case with your loved one, watch him or her carefully for signs of heat exhaustion and heat stroke. In some communities, social service agencies provide air conditioners free of charge to older people with limited incomes. Check with your local Area Agency on Aging for more information.

Many communities provide what are referred to as "cooling centers" that are open to the public throughout the summer months or during summer hot spells. Another option for keeping cool during hot weather may be a visit to a local air-conditioned shopping mall or movie theater.

Heat Exhaustion and Heatstroke

Heat exhaustion occurs when a person is exposed to a high temperature and high humidity for a prolonged period of time. Some possible symptoms of heat exhaustion include:

- Slight fever
- Excessive sweating
- Pale, clammy skin
- Dizziness, weakness, or faintness
- Headache
- Nausea
- Muscle cramps

If you notice any of these symptoms, have the person lie in a cool, quiet place with his or her feet slightly raised. Loosen any tight clothing. Give him or her cool salt water (1 level teaspoon of salt per 1 quart of water) to sip. Do not give alcohol or caffeinated beverages. Stop giving water if the person vomits. Sponge his or her forehead and body with cool water. Cool the person with a fan or move him or her to an air-conditioned room. If symptoms continue, worsen, or last for more than an hour, call for emergency medical assistance or take the person to the nearest hospital emergency department immediately.

⚠️ **WARNING:** If a person with symptoms of heat exhaustion vomits or faints, call 911 or your local emergency number, or take him or her to the nearest hospital emergency department immediately.

Heatstroke (also called sunstroke) is a life-threatening emergency caused by the body's inability to cool itself after prolonged exposure to a high temperature. Some possible symptoms of heatstroke include:

- Body temperature of 104 degrees Fahrenheit or higher
- Flushed, hot, dry skin (with no sweating)
- Rapid breathing
- Strong, rapid pulse
- Confusion
- Unconsciousness

Remove the person's clothing and sponge his or her body with cool water or rubbing alcohol until his or her temperature reaches 101 to 102 degrees Fahrenheit. Be careful not to overcool the person. Keep the person cool with a fan or move him or her to an air-conditioned room. If the person's temperature rises, begin sponging his or her body again. Call for emergency medical assistance or take the person to the nearest hospital emergency department immediately.

Depression

An older person who lives alone may feel isolated and depressed. Older people at high risk for depression are those who are ill or disabled, or who lack adequate social contact and support. Early detection and treatment of depression is extremely important because of the high risk of suicide among older people. Symptoms of depression may include feelings of guilt or apathy, loss of self-esteem, difficulty concentrating, changes in appetite (decrease or increase), weight loss or weight gain, difficulty sleeping, loss of interest in favorite activities, and a pervasive feeling of sadness. If you recognize these symptoms in your loved one, try to persuade him or her to talk to the doctor. You may also want to discuss the problem with the doctor yourself.

Some people incorrectly assume that symptoms of depression in older people are simply a normal part of aging or mistake symptoms of depression for Alzheimer's disease. For this reason, it is extremely important to have a doctor give the person a thorough evaluation. Unlike Alzheimer's disease, depression can be treated successfully with medication, psychotherapy, or a combination of both—at any age. At the same time, try not to confuse your loved one's desire for solitude or privacy with symptoms of depression. It is normal for him or her to want some privacy from time to time, and you should understand and respect this desire. Solitude provides time for a person to think, reflect, and reminisce about his or her life.

8

Caring for an Older Person Who Needs Limited Assistance

Many older people live alone and want to continue doing so for as long as possible. Caregivers should do everything possible to promote this independence. However, some older people who want to live alone require some assistance from others. Use the information in this chapter as a guide and adapt our recommendations to your loved one's particular needs and situation.

Although you have your loved one's best interests in mind, trying to make all the decisions yourself can be counterproductive. Taking over control of the person's life is likely to threaten his or her self-esteem and sense of independence. Therefore, whenever possible, encourage the person to be an active participant in making both large and small decisions, including those that involve home healthcare. Provide guidance and advice while acknowledging that the person probably prefers to have primary control over his or her life. You will be a more effective caregiver if you remember to help your loved one achieve his or her goals rather than your own.

Geriatric Care Managers

Caring for aging parents poses a special challenge for adult children who do not live nearby. In such cases, when an older person becomes physically or mentally impaired or incapacitated, it is often left to hospital personnel, such as a discharge planner or social worker, to arrange for appropriate services and continuity of care from a visiting nurse association or similar agency. After these arrangements are made, professional healthcare providers deliver skilled nursing care, physical therapy, occupational therapy, speech therapy, and any other needed services. Medicare or Medicaid often covers the cost of these services for a specified period of time. If the person's need for home healthcare extends beyond his or her Medicare benefits coverage, the services can be continued and paid for out of pocket.

Coordinating all of this care can be difficult and challenging for an older person and his or her family and is best handled by a geriatric care manager. A geriatric care manager is a social worker, nurse, or psychologist who is experienced in coordinating and overseeing the care of older people. The services that a geriatric care manager provides are designed to bring organization and stability to a difficult, potentially chaotic situation.

A geriatric care manager assumes the role of a surrogate family member and reports regularly to the person's adult children by telephone. He or she makes periodic home visits to set up, evaluate, and adjust a care plan designed to maximize the person's abilities. The care plan may include the services of a paid, direct caregiver, who may be responsible for providing or arranging transportation, housekeeping, bathing and hygiene, meal preparation, shopping, and other specified tasks. The care manager may supplement home visits with telephone calls. The effectiveness of a care plan is based in part on a good relationship between the person who is receiving care, the geriatric care manager, and the professional caregiver.

The National Association of Professional Geriatric Care Managers has a nationwide listing of professional geriatric care managers. Call them at (520) 881-8008 for more information. Costs for these services vary across the country, but, in general, you must pay for all of the services they provide, including visits, telephone calls, consultations with other agencies, supervisory visits, and interviews with professional caregivers.

If you cannot afford to hire a private geriatric care manager or if none are available in your community, call your local Area Agency on Aging, which can provide a list of organizations that offer similar services on a long-term basis. Area Agencies on Aging are usually listed in the telephone book under federal, state, or local government services.

Keeping Legal and Financial Affairs in Order

Keeping track of personal finances and important documents often becomes more difficult as a person ages. He or she may forget to make bank deposits or balance the checkbook, and bills may go unpaid. Financial and other matters may need to be managed by a family member, caregiver, geriatric care manager, or social worker, or by a lawyer who specializes in the legal and financial concerns of older people. It is important to get your loved one's affairs in order as soon as possible, ideally while he or she is still in relatively good health. This will help you avoid a frantic search for important documents after a crisis.

If your loved one is having problems keeping his or her affairs in order, you will need to gather all documents related to bank accounts, safety deposit boxes, investments, taxes, and pensions, and information about financial obligations (including bills and loans). Locate his or her Social Security and Medicare cards. Get the names and telephone numbers of all bankers, lawyers, accountants, and brokers. You will also need the names and telephone numbers of the person's doctors. Collect all other important documents such as birth certificates, life insurance policies, deeds and titles, papers relating to military service (such as discharge papers), wills, and burial arrangements. Keep all of these documents in a safe place. Have your loved one consult an attorney to prepare a living will and assign a durable power of attorney for finances and healthcare (see page 156) as soon as possible if he or she has not already done so. Also, have a lawyer prepare or review the person's will, trusts, and estate planning at this time.

Senior Centers

Senior centers often serve as a focal point of social life for older people and can provide a wide variety of needed services. In some communities, churches, hospitals, community centers, and town halls may serve the same purpose. Senior centers are available to active older people and offer a wide range of social and recreational activities as well as programs designed to promote healthy living. Some centers also provide meal programs and information and referral services for older people. Programs and services offered by senior centers are often provided free of charge or for modest fees based on a person's ability to pay.

Adult Day Care Centers

Adult day care centers have become a popular resource for older people who need assistance and supervision during the day when no one else is at home. Older people can benefit from the organized social and recreational activities that day care centers offer. Day care centers are fully equipped to provide meals and recreation and to supervise medications for older people. Field trips, parties, and other activities facilitate social interaction and help prevent the boredom that can come from a predictable daily routine. The staff members of day care centers are sensitive to the needs of older people and are usually trained to manage some health problems such as incontinence.

Adult day care is not federally regulated but may be licensed or certified by the state. Certification based on specific standards and guidelines is needed to obtain federal funding. Day care may be funded by government agencies such as Medicare, Medicaid, or the Department of Veterans Affairs. Costs are usually based on the person's income and financial resources. In some cases, day care may be covered by private insurance. The cost of attending day care is often much less per hour than the fee for a paid companion to come to the home. Ask your doctor or social worker to recommend a center in your area.

Continuing Care Retirement Communities

Continuing care retirement communities offer residents a full range of housing and care options—from independent living, to assisted living, to 24-hour skilled nursing care. Most of these communities require payment of a considerable admission fee and ongoing monthly and medical fees. These fees may increase each year. Additional fees are charged for care and services that are not covered by the monthly fees. Find out in advance which services are covered and which will require additional fees.

Services provided by continuing care retirement communities may include a specified number of meals, personal care assistance, and housekeeping. These communities usually provide recreational and social activities and may also provide on-site amenities such as a library and a hair salon. Residents may move among independent living, assisted living, and a nursing facility within the community, depending on their healthcare needs. Living in a continuing care retirement community is often too expensive for an older person with limited income and assets.

Assisted Living Facilities

Assisted living facilities are appearing in many communities throughout the United States. In an assisted living facility, older people can live in private apartments while taking advantage of many services, which may include meals in a group dining room, housekeeping, shopping trips, and general monitoring by an emergency communication system. Although there is usually no admission fee for assisted living facilities that are not part of a continuing care retirement community, monthly fees may be higher than those charged at a continuing care retirement community. Fees at assisted living facilities may increase each year, and additional fees are charged for care or services that are not covered by the monthly fee. Be sure to find out in advance which services are included and which will require additional fees.

An assisted living arrangement fosters independence while providing help with basic household management. Additional services may include the assistance of home health aides who can help with daily tasks such as getting out of bed and bathing, and provide medication reminders. These services may or may not be included in the monthly fee.

Assisted living can often help a frail older person remain independent. Some assisted living facilities have on-site nursing facilities where a resident can stay temporarily while recuperating from an illness. The person can then move back into his or her apartment after he or she has recovered.

Telephone Check-in and Reassurance

Telephone check-in and reassurance services provide a means of monitoring the health and safety of an older person who is living alone. These services are performed by paid staff or trained volunteers who call a homebound person at prearranged times throughout the day. If there is a problem or if the person does not answer the phone, the caller will follow specific procedures such as contacting a designated doctor or family member or calling for emergency assistance. These services can provide older people with companionship and a sense of security. Contact your doctor, nurse, social worker, or local hospital for information about the availability of telephone check-in and reassurance services in your area.

Area Agencies on Aging

The Older Americans Act of 1965 established a national network of federally funded state and local community service programs that are responsible for providing a wide range of services for older people. Each Area Agency on Aging provides services such as information and referrals for medical and legal services, health insurance, psychological counseling, retirement planning, abuse prevention services, shopping services, meal delivery, nutrition education programs, educational and social programs, health screening, and wellness promotion programs. To find your local Area Agency on Aging, look in your telephone book under federal, state, or local government services.

9

Providing Long-term Care

Caring for a loved one for a long period of time poses a number of challenges for any caregiver. This chapter provides useful information on dealing with the most common problems of caring for a person who is confined to bed. Prolonged inactivity can quickly lead to physical deterioration: muscles weaken, joints stiffen, and pressure sores, constipation, and problems with bowel and bladder control may develop. Inactive older people are at increased risk for thrombosis (formation of a blood clot in a blood vessel), embolism (sudden blockage of a blood vessel by a blood clot), and severe respiratory infections such as pneumonia. Confusion also seems to occur more frequently in older people who are confined to bed. Encourage your loved one to get out of bed as often as possible and to stay as active as possible.

Getting Out of Bed

A person who has been confined to bed for a long time is likely to feel weak and dizzy when getting out of bed for the first time. To prevent a fall, have the person sit up slowly and rest on the edge of the bed for a few minutes before trying to stand up. Place a sturdy chair beside the bed. When the person feels steady, stand directly in front of him or her so that he or she can lean on you for support. Hold the person under the arms. Then, help the person turn slowly, and gently and carefully lower him or her into the chair. As the person begins to feel stronger, have him or her try to take a few steps, using your arms for support. For more information about helping a person get out of bed, see page 118.

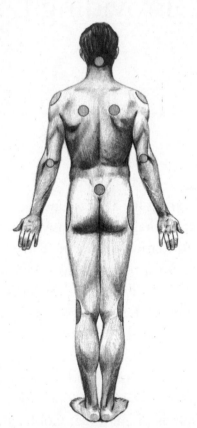

Preventing Pressure Sores

A person who is confined to bed is at risk of developing pressure sores, especially if his or her movement is restricted or sensation impaired. Pressure sores are the result of continuous pressure on certain parts of the body, which interferes with blood circulation to

Pressure Sores
Pressure sores develop on the parts of the body that bear its weight or rub against bedding. The most common sites for pressure sores are the shoulders, elbows, lower back, hips, buttocks, knees, ankles, and heels.

the tissue in the surrounding area. Poor nutrition and incontinence can also contribute to the development of pressure sores.

A pressure sore begins as a patch of tender, reddened, inflamed skin. Gradually, the skin turns purple, breaks down, and forms an open sore. The sore gradually grows larger and deeper, and often becomes infected. Pressure sores are usually very difficult and slow to heal, and will not heal at all unless pressure on the affected area is significantly reduced or eliminated.

The best way to help prevent pressure sores is to change the person's position every 2 hours when he or she is awake. Move your loved one from one side onto his or her back, then to the other side; rotate position throughout the day. It is not necessary to get up during the night specifically to turn the person, but if you are awakened for another reason, you may find it convenient to turn him or her at that time.

WARNING: Never drag a person from one position in bed to another; this could damage his or her skin and increase the risk of developing pressure sores.

Once every hour or so, have the person stimulate circulation and prevent joint stiffening by wiggling his or her toes, rotating the ankles, flexing the arms and legs, tightening and relaxing the muscles, and stretching the entire body. If the person is immobile or very weak, you can perform passive exercise by gently bending and straightening the person's joints several times each day.

Place cushions and pillows between the person's knees and under his or her shoulders to help relieve pressure. Try alternating pressure mattresses, synthetic sheepskin mattress pads, and heel protectors to allow air to circulate around the person's skin and help reduce pressure and friction against the bedding. A bed or foot cradle (a tentlike frame placed at the foot of the bed) helps to keep the weight of bedclothes off the person's feet. You can rent or purchase all of these items from drugstores and medical supply companies. In most cases, Medicare or private insurance covers the costs. Remember, however, that even when you use these items, you still need to turn the person frequently to prevent pressure sores.

Be sure to keep the sheets clean, dry, crumb free, and pulled tight to prevent wrinkles. Also, bathe the person frequently (see page 17) and keep his or her skin clean and dry, especially in those areas that are most vulnerable to pressure sores. Check the skin each day for reddening. If you see any reddening, keep pressure off the area and tell the doctor that a pressure sore appears to be forming.

Get the person out of bed as often as possible. In addition to reducing the risk of pressure sores, being active helps prevent fluid from collecting in the lungs, a major factor in the development of pneumonia. If the person cannot get out of bed, encourage him or her to move around in bed frequently. Remove soiled underwear (including disposable briefs) promptly, and wash the person's skin with warm (not hot) water and gently pat it dry with a soft towel. Gently apply alcohol-free skin cream to the skin, using a circular motion. Ask your doctor or nurse to recommend a good skin cream.

Have the person eat a healthy diet (see page 92) and drink plenty of fluids to help keep the skin healthy. Eating high-protein foods (such as lean meat, fish, dried peas and beans, and whole grains) and taking nutritional supplements can also help prevent and treat pressure sores. Nutritional supplements that provide additional nutrients and calories in a pleasant-tasting, lactose-free drink are widely available. Ask your doctor if your loved one could benefit from nutritional supplements.

Preventing the Arms and Legs from Stiffening

A period of bed rest is often required after surgery or a major illness. Encourage a person who is confined to bed for any reason to change positions frequently to prevent the joint stiffness and loss of muscle tone that can result from prolonged inactivity.

To help prevent joint stiffness, carefully place and support the person's arms and legs in comfortable, natural, strain-free positions and rest them on pillows, cushions, or pads. Rest the person's elbows on pillows, and use foam rubber cushions or pillows to keep his or her legs from turning outward. Support the person's feet with a footboard to prevent footdrop (a deformity caused by nerve damage and paralysis in certain leg muscles).

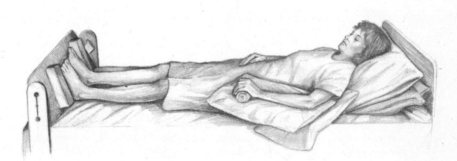

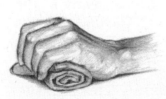

Place the person's hands around small rolls of foam rubber padding. Range-of-motion exercises will help prevent a bedridden person's arms and legs from stiffening. The person should move each of his or her limbs up and down and away from and toward the body midline. This is called active range of motion. If the person is

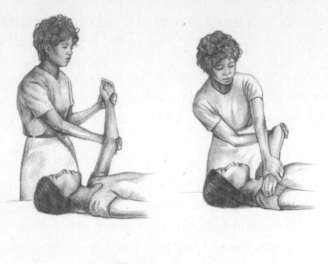

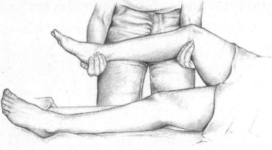

Range-of-motion Exercises
If the person you are caring for is immobile or has difficulty moving, help him or her to perform range-of-motion exercises. Gently bend and straighten each elbow and wrist, and the fingers and thumb of each hand. Raise each leg, bending and straightening the hip, knee, and ankle.

unable to move a limb, the caregiver can perform passive range of motion exercises (see above), which involve gently holding the person's limb at each joint and moving the limb in all the directions in which it can normally move. These exercises also help stimulate blood circulation and help prevent blood clots from forming in the legs. The visiting nurse will teach you how to correctly perform range-of-motion exercises. Encourage the person to move each joint through its entire range of motion several times throughout the day.

WARNING: Do not try to move any joint that resists motion. Never move any limb beyond the point at which it causes discomfort or pain. If a joint does not move easily or the person feels pain, tell the doctor as soon as possible.

Moving an Immobile Person in Bed

Moving an immobile person in bed can be challenging, and you can get seriously injured in the process. To prevent back strain, have an immobile person sleep in a hospital bed with side rails. You can raise the bed to a comfortable height, which will allow you to bathe, turn, and exercise the person without putting strain on your back. You can rent a hospital bed from a hospital supply company; Medicare usually covers about 80 percent of the cost if a doctor has prescribed the bed. To help prevent falls and serious injuries, always return the hospital bed to its lowest position each time you finish providing care.

It is easier to move a person who is very weak or immobile if you use a drawsheet (see page 27). If the person's bed does not have side rails, two caregivers need to perform this task.

STEP 1. To move the person to one side of the bed (or to turn the person on his or her side), untuck the end of the drawsheet on the opposite side of the bed.

STEP 2. Return to the side of the bed to which you want to move the person.

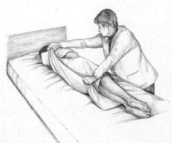

STEP 3. Reach over the person, gather the drawsheet in your hands at the person's hip and shoulder area, and gently roll the person toward you.

STEP 4. Smooth out and tuck in the drawsheet.

A person who is confined to bed may have a tendency to slide toward the foot of the bed. To move an immobile person toward the head of the bed, you first need to help him or her to a sitting position.

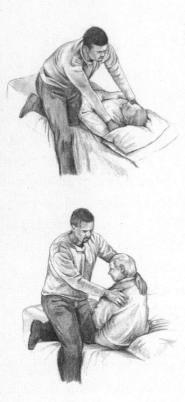

STEP 1.   To help a person sit up in bed, first arrange the pillows so that his or her shoulders are elevated. Cross the person's arms and rest them at his or her waist. Place your hands over the person's shoulders and place your knee on the bed, next to his or her hip. Place your other foot firmly on the floor next to the bed, slightly ahead of your knee and even with the person's waist.

STEP 2.   Firmly grasp the person's shoulders, keeping your arms straight, and slowly sit back, using your weight to pull him or her up toward you.

STEP 3.   If you want to move the person toward the head of the bed, keep your hand on the shoulder closest to you and get in position behind him or her. Place your knee on the bed behind the person and place your other foot firmly on the floor. Cross the person's forearms in front of his or her waist and hold them firmly

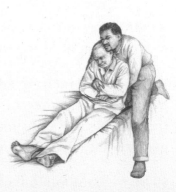

from behind. Slowly sit back, using your weight to pull the person toward you.

You can also use a drawsheet to move a person up in bed, but you will need help from another caregiver to safely perform this task.

STEP 1. Caregivers should stand at opposite sides of the bed.

STEP 2. Untuck both ends of the drawsheet (each caregiver untucks one end).

STEP 3. Grasp both ends of the drawsheet (each caregiver grasps one end) and carefully lift the person toward the head of the bed.

Positioning an Immobile Person in Bed

Always position an immobile person's body in proper alignment to help prevent the arms and legs from stiffening. You can do this using pillows and bolsters. For example, when a person is lying on his or her side, instead of elevating the head of the bed, place a pillow under the upper leg and arm. And place a pillow or bolster behind the person's back to prevent him or her from rolling backward. A person who has little flesh on the hips should not be positioned fully on his or her side. Instead, position him or her in a 30-degree side-lying position (see illustration on next page). This will help prevent pressure and the development of pressure sores in the hip area.

An immobile person who is confined to bed should not remain in the same position for longer than 2 hours while the caregiver is awake. Move the person from his or her side, onto his or her back, and onto his or her other side every 2 hours. When the immobile person is on his or her back, place a pillow

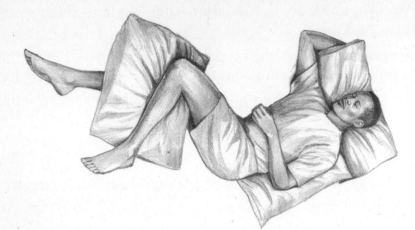

under each arm and on the side of each thigh to prevent the hips from rotating outward. Also, place a small pillow under the knees and a footboard at the foot of the bed to keep the person's feet positioned at a right angle to the mattress. This will prevent footdrop (a deformity caused by nerve damage and paralysis in certain leg muscles) and keep the person from sliding down the bed. Do not tuck sheets and blankets tightly around the person's feet and legs; keep the bedclothes loose with a bed or foot cradle (a tentlike frame placed at the foot of the bed). Keep bottom sheets taut to prevent wrinkles and pressure under the body, which could cause pressure sores.

When feeding a person in bed, elevate the head of the bed at least 30 degrees to prevent choking. And keep the bed raised for at least an hour after eating. This helps prevent regurgitation of food, which can lead to aspiration (accidentally breathing a solid or liquid into the lungs) and subsequent choking or development of pneumonia.

Transferring an Immobile Person

In general, transferring an immobile person requires both physical strength and training. Without proper training, a caregiver can easily injure his or her back while trying to move a person from a bed to a chair or wheelchair. A nurse or physical therapist can train you in the proper technique. When transferring an immobile person, wear sturdy shoes with nonskid soles and make sure that the person you are transferring is also wearing sturdy, nonskid shoes or slippers. To help prevent falls, do not attempt to transfer a person who is barefoot or wearing only socks. You may need to use a transfer belt, a specially designed belt that you place around the immobile person's waist. The belt provides leverage and makes it easier to firmly grip the person when you help him or her to a standing or sitting position. Ask your doctor, nurse, or home health aide to show you how to use a transfer belt properly. You can purchase one from a medical supply company.

⚠️ **WARNING:** Never substitute another type of belt for a transfer belt when moving an immobile person; you could cause serious injury to the person.

Before you begin:

- If you are transferring the person from a hospital bed, lock the bed's brakes.
- If you are transferring the person to a wheelchair, lock the wheelchair's brakes.
- If needed, put a transfer belt on the person.
- Tell the person what you are going to do before you begin each step.

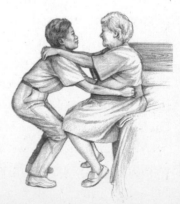

STEP 1. Carefully assist the person to a sitting position on the side of the bed with his or her feet on the floor. If the person has been confined to bed for a long time, allow

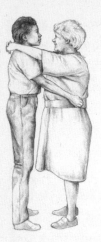

him or her to rest on the edge of the bed until he or she feels secure. Stand directly in front of the person and brace his or her knees with your knees. Carefully slide his or her hips toward you.

STEP 2.   Help the person to a standing position, using the transfer belt if necessary, while firmly holding him or her around the waist.

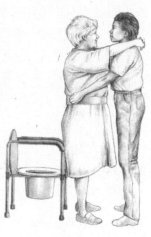

STEP 3.   Slowly pivot the person around until his or her back is directly in front of the chair, wheelchair, or commode; have the person feel the seat of the chair or commode with the back of his or her legs before attempting to sit.

STEP 4.   Slowly lower the person to a sitting position. Once he or she is seated securely, remove the transfer belt.

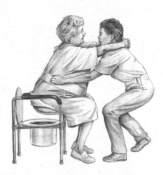

To help the person back to bed, perform the steps described above in reverse order. Be sure to lock the brakes on the bed and wheelchair before you begin, and use the transfer belt. If you are using a hospital bed, be sure to raise the bed rails after the person is back in bed.

Mechanical lifts, which are used to transfer an immobile person easily and safely, are available from medical supply companies. One type works with hydraulic pressure, which enables one caregiver to safely transfer a completely paralyzed person weighing up to 400 pounds. The medical supply company will teach you how to use the lift. Medicare or other third-party insurers usually cover the cost of a lift if it has been prescribed by a doctor.

Dealing with Memory Problems

Memory problems are sometimes related to aging. Normal memory problems may include forgetting to call a relative on his or her birthday or leaving some of the ingredients out of a favorite recipe. People of all ages have these types of memory problems and they don't interfere with their ability to function. When an older person realizes that his or her memory is not as good as it once was, he or she may begin to feel apprehensive, fearful, and anxious. Forgetfulness may cause an older person to assume that he or she is developing Alzheimer's disease. Reassure the person and try the following strategies to help him or her remember better:

- Make signs to remind the person to do things such as take medication, turn off the stove, or lock the doors. Place them in a visible location.
- Give the person a large calendar with large numbers to help him or her keep track of dates and events by checking off each day of the week.
- Circle dates on the calendar as a reminder of important appointments and dates.
- Provide clocks with large, easy-to-read numbers to help the person stay time-oriented.
- Follow a regular mealtime schedule; people with memory problems often forget to eat.

- Post a daily checklist on the refrigerator door to remind the person of the things he or she needs to do.
- Place items to bring upstairs on a table near the foot of the stairs (but never on the stairs).
- Place items to be taken along on outings on a table near the front door.
- Label boxes with their contents so the person will know at a glance what's inside.
- Store items such as keys, eyeglasses, and medications in the same place so that they are easy to find when needed. Be sure to always return them to their proper place.
- If the person is disoriented, have him or her wear an identification bracelet at all times; it should list his or her name, address, and telephone number and the name and number of someone to contact. This will be helpful if he or she wanders away or becomes lost.

Some senior centers offer memory-enhancing classes to help older people improve their ability to remember. If your loved one's memory problems begin to interfere with day-to-day living, he or she should be examined by a doctor who has experience diagnosing and treating people with Alzheimer's disease. For information about Alzheimer's disease, see chapter 11.

10

Nursing Homes

No matter how good a caregiver you are, it may eventually become necessary to consider placing your loved one in a nursing home or some other chronic care facility. The decision is never easy to make, and the issue is often emotionally charged and very personal. For some families, the decision is made gradually, as the person's condition declines and it becomes evident that he or she needs special care, or as caregiving tasks become more and more difficult to perform. For other families, however, the decision is made quickly, under very stressful circumstances.

Placing a loved one in a nursing home may cause him or her to feel abandoned or angry. He or she may feel heartbroken after losing independence and at the thought of leaving his or her home and possessions, and losing his or her privacy and, perhaps, dignity. The person may fear losing contact with family and friends. The caregiver may experience similar concerns and fears, along with feelings of loneliness, ineffectiveness, and guilt. Everyone involved may also be worried about financial matters: how much will this cost and how will we pay for it?

On the other hand, choosing to place your loved one in a nursing home may also bring feelings of relief to everyone concerned. In addition to providing more complete care, such settings can provide residents with new friends and experiences. Loved ones may take comfort in knowing they have lessened the caregiver's burden, and the relationship may become less strained as a result.

Deciding What Is Best for Your Loved One and You

Before you make this difficult decision, evaluate the situation by asking some important questions and providing some honest answers. Be realistic. Do not deceive yourself or let feelings of guilt interfere with an honest appraisal of your options. Some questions to ask when considering whether to allow your loved one to remain at home or place him or her in a nursing home or other chronic care facility include the following:

- Does the person need 24-hour care or supervision? Is skilled care required? Can the type and level of care needed be provided at home?
- How much assistance with activities of daily living does the person require? Will these needs increase over time? Can they be met at home?
- Are you, the caregiver, capable of providing the appropriate level and quality of care and attention?

Do not make this decision lightly—or alone. Involve your loved one as well as other family members and members of the caregiving team—doctors, nurses, social workers, discharge planners, close friends, and members of the clergy. Though discussions may be difficult and at times painful, addressing these sensitive issues directly and early in the process may help prevent other problems in the future. If you are the primary caregiver and family members want the person to stay at home, be direct and firm in asking the family members what they can contribute in terms of time or money.

Choosing a Nursing Home

Once you have decided to place your loved one in a nursing home or other chronic care facility, you must carefully choose the best place possible. After selecting an appropriate facility, have an attorney review and explain all relevant documents before you sign a contract, to make sure that you are aware of your rights and obligations under the law. This will help to prevent future disputes or misunderstandings.

Your decision should be based on complete and accurate information. Here are some important factors to consider and questions to ask when looking for an appropriate nursing home for your loved one:

- If possible, get recommendations from friends, relatives, clergy, or your doctor or other members of the caregiving team.

- Limit your choices according to significant factors such as size, location, cost, and religious affiliation.

- Visit the facilities that meet your criteria. Stay long enough at each to form an opinion about the general atmosphere of the facility (does it seem friendly and relaxed or rigid and tense?) and to meet on site with residents, administrators, and caregivers. Try to visit at mealtimes to get a realistic impression of the facility at work.

- Contact your state licensing board to determine how the nursing home is rated, how it fares on inspections, and whether any complaints have been filed, and if so, the nature of the complaints.

- Find out who owns the facility and who is on its board of directors. Also, find out the facility's hospital affiliations. Is the facility accredited by the Joint Commission on Accreditation of Healthcare Organizations?

- Are potential staff members given criminal background checks prior to hiring?

- Does the staff include people who have the skills your loved one may need, including registered nurses, licensed practical nurses, nurses' aides, and a physician or medical director (either on call 24 hours or on site). What is the rate of staff turnover?

- Can your loved one continue to see his or her own doctor, or will he or she be required to see a doctor who is affiliated with the nursing home?

- What are the nursing home's emergency procedures? Which ambulance service and hospital emergency department are used in case of a medical emergency? What is the facility's policy for notifying loved ones in case of an emergency?

- What are the facility's policies regarding the use of restraints? Federal law allows the use of physical restraints (such as belts, vests, or raised bed rails) and chemical restraints (such as tranquilizers and sedatives) on nursing facility residents only for clear medical reasons or to protect other residents of the facility. Except in emergencies, restraints cannot be used without written orders from a physician.

- Does the facility accept younger patients with chronic illnesses such as mental disorders? If so, are these patients separated from the other residents?

- What are the staff-to-resident ratio, the level of care given around the clock, and the types of skilled personnel—including physical and occupational therapists, recreation directors, dietitians, social workers, and members of the clergy—that are available to residents?

- Does the food look appetizing and taste good? Are dining rooms provided for residents? Do residents receive adequate assistance with meals if they cannot feed themselves? Can the facility accommodate your loved one's special dietary needs, such as a low-sodium or kosher diet?

- What is the physical condition of the nursing home? Does it look like a comfortable place? Are the rooms, stairways, and hallways well lit? Does everything appear to be clean and in good repair? Are there any unpleasant odors? Does the facility smell of urine?

- What is the toilet policy? Do staff members routinely place residents who wear absorbent disposable briefs on the toilet at specific intervals?

- What extra services—such as personal grooming services, laundry, a recreation room, and a library—are provided? Which services are included in the contract, and which ones cost extra? Who is responsible for the cost of prescriptions, medical equipment and supplies, television, telephone, or outside activities?

- Can residents' rooms be personalized? Is the room size adequate? How many residents are assigned to each room? Can residents change rooms? Are single rooms available?

- Are private shower or bath facilities provided?

- Do the residents' rooms and bathrooms have safety features such as handrails, grab bars, and emergency call buttons?

- What is the nursing home's policy regarding theft of personal property? What does the facility do to prevent theft of residents' personal property? Is theft covered by insurance?

- Is it easy for residents to get to their rooms or other areas of the facility? Where are the nursing stations located?

- What types of recreational activities are available? How often are they offered? Are these activities also tailored to the needs of residents with dementia?

- Are residents permitted to go outdoors? Are the grounds safe and secure?

- Does the nursing home actively encourage visitors?

- Do clergy members pay regular visits to residents? Are religious services offered? For which denominations are they available?

- What are the facility's fees and how will finances be handled? Does the facility meet government guidelines for Medicare and Medicaid coverage? What costs are covered by Medicare, Medicaid, or private insurance?

- What is the nursing home's deposit and refund policy? If the cost of your loved one's care will be covered by Medicare or Medicaid, a nursing home cannot require you to pay a cash deposit prior to admission. Federal law prohibits prepayment of fees by Medicare and Medicaid beneficiaries. However, a nursing home can require a cash deposit for potential residents who are not covered by Medicare or Medicaid.

Your local long-term care ombudsman is often a good resource for the type of information you need to help you choose a nursing home in your area. Although a long-term care ombudsman cannot recommend specific nursing homes, he or she can provide you with useful information about such crucial factors as quality of care, quality of life, results of state inspections, and the number and types of complaints, if any. To locate the long-term care ombudsman for your area, contact your Area Agency on Aging, listed in the telephone book under federal, state, or local government services.

Monitoring Your Loved One's Care

Once your loved one moves into a nursing home, it is extremely important to visit regularly and continually monitor his or her condition and quality of life. Be especially observant about the following:

- **Personal appearance.** Does your loved one look clean and well groomed? Are his or her clothes clean? Check for pressure sores and bruises. Also check for wet or soiled disposable briefs.

- **Food service.** Are meals served on time and at the proper temperature? Are special dietary needs being met? Are serving sizes adequate? If the person requires assistance to eat, is this help being provided?

- **Room condition.** Is the bedding changed frequently? Is the room cleaned at regular intervals?

- **Staff.** Are staff members friendly and helpful? Are they available to answer your questions? Do they respond to requests from you and your loved one? Do they contact you whenever significant changes occur, such as in medical treatment or in your loved one's condition? Do they respect your loved one's privacy?

- **Other residents.** Do they seem to be alert, content, and well cared for? Does your loved one get along well with his or her roommate?

In addition to your own observations, ask your loved one about the care he or she receives, and how he or she feels about the care at the nursing home. The more contact you have with your loved one and the nursing home, the better you can monitor the care he or she receives. Talk to some of the other residents and find out how they feel about the nursing home and the care that they receive. Talk to staff members, too. It is a good idea to visit the nursing home unannounced, especially at night and on weekends.

If you suspect that your loved one is receiving less-than-adequate care or is being abused in any way, respond cautiously but decisively. Document your loved one's complaints as well as your own concerns. If the problems are merely a matter of misunderstanding or oversight, then having a clear discussion with the nursing home's ombudsman, administrator, or staff should resolve the situation. It may be helpful to follow up such communication in writing, outlining your concerns and your understanding of how the matter will be handled. You may also want to report any concerns you may have about the treatment of other residents of the nursing home.

It is important to note that some residents of nursing homes may be hesitant to report problems because they do not want family members or nursing home staff to think they are chronic complainers or troublemakers. They may also fear punishment, whether real or imagined. Consequently, some problems that should be resolved may go unreported. On the other hand, some residents may complain about staff or roommates because they feel they are not getting enough attention from family members, or for other reasons.

Sometimes the people who live in a nursing home work together to deal with issues that concern them by forming and participating in a resident council. The council meets on a regular basis to identify and discuss various problems and concerns of residents and to develop and offer possible solutions. If such a group exists in your loved one's nursing home, it may provide the easiest forum for him or her to resolve any problems or misunderstandings about his or her experiences in the facility. Participating in council meetings can provide needed support and a constructive way to express concerns and resolve problems without the fear of getting into trouble for complaining.

If there are serious problems that remain unresolved, it may be necessary to contact the local or state public health department, the state regulatory or licensing agency for nursing homes, an accrediting agency such as the Joint Commission on Accreditation of Healthcare Organizations, or local chapters of consumer advocacy groups. In cases of abuse or neglect, the matter must be reported to the police.

Paying for Care in a Nursing Home

Although fees vary somewhat across the United States, the cost of care in a nursing home is usually high. Half of the people who live in nursing homes pay for their care with savings and other assets. If a person's stay in the nursing home is lengthy and depletes most or all of his or her assets, he or she usually becomes eligible to receive Medicaid coverage. Managed care plans, such as health maintenance organizations, do not cover the costs of long-term care.

Medicaid

Medicaid is a state program financed with state and federal funds that provides medical insurance for low-income residents. In general, the program covers most of the costs of care in a Medicaid-certified nursing facility. Eligibility requirements and benefits vary from state to state. Contact your local Medicaid office for additional information.

Medicare

Medicare is a federal program that provides medical insurance for people who are 65 years of age and over, have a disability, or have end-stage kidney disease. Medicare will cover some of the costs of care in a Medicare-certified nursing facility when specific requirements are met. For information about Medicare eligibility and benefits, call the Social Security Administration at (800) 772-1213, or contact the Health Care Financing Administration at (800) MEDICARE (633-4227).

Medicare Supplemental Insurance

Medicare supplemental insurance (sometimes called Medigap insurance) is private insurance that may pay for care in a nursing home if that care is also covered by Medicare. In general, these policies are designed to cover the costs of short-term care only, such as recovery from an injury, major surgery, or acute illness; they do not cover the costs of long-term care. Review your policy or contact your insurer for additional information.

Long-term Care Insurance

Long-term care insurance may cover some of the costs of care in a nursing home. Long-term care insurance is usually available only to people who are in generally good health at the time they purchase the policy. Coverage varies considerably from one policy to another. For information on eligibility and benefits, check your policy or contact your insurer.

11

Caring for a Person Who Has Alzheimer's Disease

Alzheimer's disease is an incurable condition of unknown cause in which nerve cells in the brain degenerate and die, causing progressive memory loss, confusion, physical deterioration, and, eventually, death. Alzheimer's disease is the most common cause of irreversible dementia (progressive deterioration of mental functioning) and most frequently occurs in people over age 65. As the disease progresses, the person becomes more confused and experiences personality and behavior changes. He or she will need more and more care, which can become increasingly difficult and exhausting for the caregiver. Keeping a positive perspective and good sense of humor can help you cope with the challenging times ahead.

While there is no cure for Alzheimer's disease at this time, medications are available that help slow the progression of the disease and manage some of the behavior problems that may accompany it. Two drugs that have been approved by the US Food and Drug Administration (FDA) to treat Alzheimer's disease—donepezil hydrochloride and tacrine—may help relieve symptoms of Alzheimer's disease in some people and help them maintain their ability to perform activities of daily living, such as eating, bathing, dressing, and using the toilet. Other potential drugs for treating Alzheimer's disease are currently under investigation.

Learning about the Disease

As a caregiver, the best thing you can do is to educate yourself so that you know what to expect and what will be expected of you. Although caring for a loved one who has Alzheimer's disease is demanding and stressful, there are a number of things you can do to prepare yourself to deal realistically with this difficult situation:

- Watch your loved one carefully to detect early warning signs of Alzheimer's disease, such as forgetfulness, irritability, and loss of interest in his or her usual daily activities (see next page).
- Gather helpful information—such as educational materials and referrals to support groups—from your local chapter of the Alzheimer's Association.
- Take all necessary safety precautions to protect your loved one from potential dangers such as burns, falls, poisoning, and wandering away from home (see page 137).
- Make all necessary legal and financial arrangements as soon as possible, including advance directives (see page 156) and payment of healthcare costs.
- Be realistic about the inevitable outcome of the disease and prepare yourself to make informed decisions about long-term care (see chapter 9).
- Take care of yourself (see chapter 13).
- Seek help and support from others who understand your situation.

Alzheimer's disease is divided into three stages: early, middle, and late. Being aware of the various stages of the disease makes it easier for caregivers to know what to expect and to develop a useful care plan that is tailored to the person's specific needs. A number of excellent books are available, especially for family caregivers, that have been written by experts on Alzheimer's disease. Ask your doctor to recommend one, or check with your local librarian. You may also contact the Alzheimer's Association Benjamin B. Green-Field Library & Resource Center (see page 188) or your local chapter of the Alzheimer's Association for books, journals, and other resources on Alzheimer's disease.

Is It Alzheimer's? Ten Warning Signs

To help you recognize the warning signs of Alzheimer's disease, the Alzheimer's Association has developed a checklist of common symptoms. (Some of these symptoms may also apply to other forms of dementia.) Review the list and check the symptoms that concern you. If you make several marks, the person who has the symptoms should see a physician for a complete examination.

1. *Recent memory loss that affects job skills.*   It is normal to occasionally forget assignments, colleagues' names, or a business associate's telephone number, then remember them later. People who have dementia, such as Alzheimer's disease, may forget things more often, and not remember them later.

2. *Difficulty performing familiar tasks.*   Busy people can be so distracted from time to time that they may leave the carrots on the stove and not remember to serve them until the end of the meal. People with Alzheimer's disease could prepare a meal and forget not only to serve it but also that they prepared it.

3. *Problems with language.*   Everyone has trouble finding the right word sometimes, but a person with Alzheimer's disease may forget simple words or substitute inappropriate words, making what he or she says incomprehensible.

4. *Disorientation of time and place.*   It is normal to forget the day of the week or your destination for a moment. But people with Alzheimer's disease can become lost on their own street, not knowing where they are, how they got there, or how to get back home.

5. *Poor or decreased judgment.*   People can become so immersed in an activity that they forget for a moment about the child they're watching. People with Alzheimer's disease may forget entirely about the child under their care. They may also dress inappropriately, such as wearing an overcoat on a hot day or wearing several shirts or blouses at once.

6. *Problems with abstract thinking.*   Balancing a checkbook may be difficult for anyone when the task is more complicated than usual. A person with Alzheimer's disease may forget completely what the numbers are and what needs to be done with them.

7. *Misplacing things.*   Anyone can temporarily misplace a wallet or keys. A person with Alzheimer's disease may put things in inappropriate places, such as an iron in the freezer or a wristwatch in the sugar bowl.

8. *Changes in mood or behavior.*   Everyone becomes sad or moody from time to time. A person with Alzheimer's disease can exhibit rapid mood swings—from calm to tears to anger—for no apparent reason.

9. *Changes in personality.*   People's personalities ordinarily change somewhat with age. But a person with Alzheimer's disease can change drastically, becoming extremely confused, suspicious, or fearful.

10. *Loss of initiative.*   It is normal to get bored with housework, a job, or social obligations from time to time, but most people soon regain their initiative. A person with Alzheimer's disease may become very passive for long periods and require cues and prompting to become involved.

Safety

Some steps you as a caregiver can take toward maintaining a safe environment are helpful for a person at any stage of Alzheimer's disease. Safety is always an issue, because a person with Alzheimer's disease often does not have the judgment to act in his or her own best interests.

Home Safety

As a caregiver, you are challenged to provide the safest possible environment and at the same time foster the person's independence. You must do all you can to protect the person while resisting the urge to overprotect him or her. It may be difficult to achieve this balance, but it is important to ensure that the person's self-image and self-esteem remain intact.

Here are some useful tips to help ensure your and your loved one's safety:

- Purchase a fire extinguisher and make sure that everyone in the household knows how to use it and maintain it.

- Carefully store all hazardous objects and materials, such as firearms, knives, paint, drain opener, and cleaning fluids. It is best to keep these types of items securely locked away and inaccessible to the person.

- Keep all medications (including over-the-counter drugs) and alcohol locked away, and dispose of all expired medications. This will help prevent poisoning or accidental overdosing.

- Cover all radiators, remove all matches and lighters, and set the water heater to below 110 degrees Fahrenheit. This will help prevent burns.

- If the person tries to use the stove, consider removing the knobs and storing them in a secure place.

- Install dead-bolt locks that require a key to open outside doors from the inside. This will help to prevent the person from wandering away from home. But make sure that the key is readily accessible in case of fire or other emergency. Also, check to make sure that this type of lock is legal in your community. Consider installing special locks on the windows and on doors that lead to attics and basements. Install an alarm system on outside doors. Sometimes, putting a STOP or KEEP OUT sign on the inside of exterior doors prevents a person with Alzheimer's disease from opening those doors. Put away essential items for going out, such as a coat or purse.

- Install smoke detectors and carbon monoxide detectors and check them regularly to make sure that they are in good working order. Replace batteries once a year on a special day, such as a birthday.

- Make sure that lighting throughout the house or apartment is sufficient to prevent shadows on the walls. Hallways and stairways should be well lit, and night-lights should be strategically placed along the route from the bedroom to the bathroom and in the bathroom itself.

- Make sure all carpeting lies flat and secure, including carpeting on stairs. Remove all throw rugs. Do not wax tile or linoleum floors. Place nonskid mats in the bathroom and kitchen.

- Avoid moving furniture around or using furniture with wheels. Keep floors and stairways free of clutter. Place electrical and phone cords close to walls.

- To help prevent the person from accidentally urinating in closets or elsewhere in the house, put a clearly marked sign on the bathroom door.
- Cover or remove mirrors if the reflections pose a threat to the person.

First-aid Kit

Organize a first-aid kit that contains the following basic items:
- Adhesive tape and bandages
- Gauze
- Elastic bandage
- Sling
- Disposable latex gloves
- Cotton balls
- Scissors
- Tweezers
- Safety pins
- Thermometer (not glass; the electronic ear-insertion type may be the best choice)
- Disposable cold packs
- Antiseptic wipes
- Antibiotic cream
- Hydrogen peroxide (3 percent solution) or rubbing alcohol
- Soap
- Calamine lotion
- Syrup of ipecac (to treat poisoning)
- Activated charcoal (to treat poisoning)
- Aspirin and acetaminophen tablets
- Flashlight
- A first-aid manual, such as the *American Medical Association Handbook of First Aid and Emergency Care*

Store the first-aid kit in a convenient location and return it to the same place after each use. Check the contents of the kit at regular intervals so that you can replace items that have been used up or whose expiration date has passed.

Finding a Loved One Who Wanders Off

Some people with Alzheimer's disease may wander away from home. Constant vigilance is your first line of defense. Taking the steps mentioned on page 138, such as installing dead-bolt locks on outside doors, can help prevent the person from wandering. It is also a good idea to ask your neighbors to call you immediately if they see your loved one alone outdoors.

However, even when you have taken every precaution to prevent your loved one from wandering, he or she may still manage to wander off and become lost. You can do a number of things to help locate and identify your loved one if he or she becomes lost. First, obtain an identification bracelet or necklace that clearly identifies the person and his or her condition. This will allow him or her to be identified readily. The Alzheimer's Association has a program called Safe Return, which provides identification for people with memory problems. The material the program provides includes a bracelet or necklace, clothing labels, and a wallet identification card. It is also a good idea to have a recent photograph of the person in case the police need to search for him or her. Unwashed clothing with the person's scent will help specially trained dogs track the person during a search, if necessary.

Safe Return maintains a nationwide 24-hour, toll-free number to call when someone is either lost or found. This service can be especially helpful if you are traveling with your loved one and are far from home when he or she wanders off. The program provides access to approximately 17,000 law enforcement agencies throughout the United States. When you report a lost person to Safe Return, you receive guidance on searching the area and contacting the police to report the person missing. The program also recommends ways to ensure that a person who has a memory problem carries or wears his or her identification at all times. Contact the Alzheimer's Association at (800) 272-3900 for more information about the Safe Return program.

Recreational Activities

To enhance the quality of your loved one's life, try to engage him or her in recreational activities, which may also help to decrease agitation or behavioral problems. Regular exercise can help to minimize feelings of restlessness, which may, in turn, help prevent wandering. It is important to coordinate these activities with the person's changing abilities during each stage of the disease. Plan activities that give the person some sense of accomplishment and satisfaction. You don't want him or her to feel frustrated or incompetent. Schedule activities for when the person is well rested and agreeable.

Before beginning any recreational activity, give basic instructions by breaking each activity into smaller steps. Talk the person through each step in a calm, gentle voice, and offer him or her appropriate praise and encouragement. If the person becomes agitated or upset, do not attempt to force him or her to continue. As the disease progresses, engage the person in uncomplicated activities. For example, you might want to try having the person paint a picture, draw, color, or use modeling clay. Play simple card games with the person, do a jigsaw puzzle, look at old photographs, or just sit and listen to calming music. Whenever possible, give the person easy meal-preparation tasks, such as washing vegetables or folding napkins. Activities should always be dignified and appropriate for adults.

Everyday activities (such as washing dishes, doing laundry, making beds, folding towels, sweeping floors, and dusting) are often easy for a peson with Alzheimer's disease to do because he or she did them before the onset of the disease.

Encouraging the person to perform these and similar helpful tasks will reinforce his or her feeling of usefulness and accomplishment.

Early-Stage Alzheimer's Disease

At the early stage of Alzheimer's disease, your loved one may develop behavior and personality changes, become forgetful, and have difficulty dealing with his or her usual activities. Family members and friends may notice subtle changes at first, but may attribute these changes to stress, loneliness, depression, or normal aging. In many cases, family members seek a diagnosis only when they can no longer cope with the person's behavior problems. If you notice any of these changes in a loved one or friend, gently persuade him or her to talk to a physician. It is very important to obtain a diagnosis to rule out other illnesses that are treatable. If the physician says your family member has mild dementia, and not Alzheimer's disease, the information in this section should still be helpful to you.

Your goal as caregiver is to help maintain the person's self-esteem and functional independence for as long as possible. Focus on what the person can do rather than on what he or she cannot do. However, as your loved one's critical thinking and judgment become more and more impaired, you may need to make changes to ensure his or her safety and the safety of others. For example, you may need to supervise medications, take the person's car keys, and curtail some activities, such as cooking or baby-sitting.

Driving

Driving often presents problems for people with dementia. Even after a confirmed diagnosis of Alzheimer's disease, many people want to continue driving and do not believe there is an urgent need to stop. For many people, driving is strongly connected with their self-esteem and sense of independence. A diagnosis of Alzheimer's disease does not mean that the person has automatically lost the ability to drive; however, safety must always be the main consideration. Caregivers should continually evaluate the person to determine if it is safe for him or her to drive.

One way to try to convince your loved one to stop driving is to request a statement from the doctor declaring that the person is no longer able to drive. If this does not work, take more direct action. In some cases, hiding the car keys may be effective. You may need to remove the distributor cap or battery from the engine to disable the car. You might also ask the doctor to write a "do not drive" prescription and take it to your local department of motor vehicles. This will help to ensure that the state is aware of the problem. Legal restrictions often are the most effective deterrent to driving.

Medication

A person with Alzheimer's disease cannot be trusted to take medication correctly. Errors in taking medication can be eliminated by taking all prescription and nonprescription medications away from the person and having them administered by the caregiver. Medications that are injected (such as insulin for a person with diabetes) can be especially challenging for a caregiver. Also, problems can develop when a person cannot express when he or she is experiencing serious symptoms as a result of an illness or side effects from a medication (such as a low blood sugar reaction). Insulin shock can occur if a person has not eaten sufficient food to balance the insulin he or she has been given. Therefore, the caregiver must take extra care to ensure that a person with diabetes and Alzheimer's disease follows an appropriate diet and is carefully monitored for a low or high blood-sugar reaction. For general information about dealing with medication, see page 95.

Financial and Legal Matters

A person with early-stage Alzheimer's disease will begin at some point to have problems taking care of his or her personal affairs. He or she may have difficulty balancing a checkbook and may forget to deposit checks and pay bills. He or she may misplace important documents, such as tax returns or bank statements. However, as long as a person with Alzheimer's disease is mentally competent, you should include him or her in all legal, financial, and healthcare decisions that relate to him or her. A mentally competent person can also indicate preferences for end-of-life care and designate a person to make decisions when he or she is no longer able to do so.

Eventually, your loved one will not be competent to make decisions about his or her finances or healthcare. When this occurs, you should hand over control of legal, financial, and medical decisions to a designated family member, friend, guardian, or attorney who will act in the person's best interests. For information about handling your loved one's legal and financial affairs and making medical decisions, see page 104.

Diet and Nutrition

Following a healthy diet can be a challenge for a person with Alzheimer's disease. Physical problems, when combined with impaired memory and judgment, can pose serious health and safety risks, especially if the person prepares his or her own meals. These risks include burns and fire caused by hot or unattended pots, pans, and burners; falls caused by slipping on spilled food or water or climbing up to reach overhead cupboards; and food poisoning caused by improperly stored or prepared foods. The person may have a poor appetite, or may simply forget to eat, even if he or she receives home-delivered meals. In some cases, the person may eat all of the delivered meals at one time and not have any food left for the rest of the day.

In regard to these potential problems, it is the caregiver's responsibility to ensure that the person eats a balanced diet. The caregiver can prepare the person's meals, designate another dependable person to prepare them, or arrange to have meals delivered to the home. In any case, the caregiver needs to make sure that the person actually eats. You may be able to do this by simple observation, but you may also want to weigh the person on a regular basis to watch for any weight loss. People with Alzheimer's disease frequently lose weight at this stage because they simply forget to eat.

General Healthcare

A person with Alzheimer's disease may live 20 years or more from the time initial symptoms develop. Because the course of the disease can be prolonged, it is vital to take steps to maintain the person's physical health, including regular physical examinations. Your loved one should have a baseline evaluation of his or her eyesight soon after the diagnosis of Alzheimer's disease; if eyeglasses need to be changed, this is the time to do it. His or her hearing should also be checked at this time. The reason for prompt action in taking care of the person's vision and hearing is that later in the course of the disease he or she will not be able to answer the questions commonly asked during vision and hearing examinations.

It is also important for the person to see a dentist at this time to ensure that his or her teeth and gums are healthy and to have necessary dental work performed as soon as possible. It is much more difficult to perform dental work on a person with middle-stage Alzheimer's disease than it is in the early stage, and preventive dental care can help reduce problems as the disease progresses.

Social Changes

Some caregivers may mistakenly believe that a person with Alzheimer's disease is able to control many of the symptoms of the disease. A person with early-stage Alzheimer's disease may still be able to respond appropriately in social situations. But he or she may feel embarrassed, fearful, and apprehensive about the changes he or she is experiencing and may try very hard to conceal any inadequacies. He or she may eventually refuse to interact with others and may withdraw and become isolated and depressed. It may be helpful to have the person seek counseling or join a support group so that he or she can share his or her feelings and experiences with other people who are at this stage of the disease.

During the early stage of the disease, you may want to encourage your loved one to continue enjoying his or her usual activities, but always consider safety first. For example, any activity that requires power tools or driving requires a certain level of skill and judgment and, therefore, should not be pursued. Activities such as walking, watching videos, or playing cards are better choices.

Emotions

While Alzheimer's disease erodes memory and results in increasing confusion, it is important for caregivers to remember that the person still has feelings. He or she may feel more or less emotional than in the past but can still respond to emotions such as anger and love and can sense when people are either angry or loving. In fact, anger in a caregiver usually generates agitation and aggression in a person with Alzheimer's disease.

Middle-Stage Alzheimer's Disease

The middle stage of Alzheimer's disease presents many additional challenges for the affected person and his or her caregiver. During this stage, your loved one may develop behavior problems such as agitation, aggression, pacing, wandering, hallucinations, overreactions to insignificant events, and worsening of behavior late in the day (referred to as sundowning). The person may have difficulty bathing, eating, or sleeping. He or she may also have delusions or paranoia or exhibit inappropriate sexual behavior.

Communication

Your loved one may have a problem finding the right words to express himself or herself and, in some cases, may make up words. He or she may also have difficulty understanding conversations and may withdraw as a response. The key to successful communication is to keep it simple and direct. Here are some helpful tips for promoting good communication:

- Eliminate distractions such as television and radio when you are talking to the person.
- Speak slowly and clearly.
- Keep your voice low and calm.
- Use simple sentences that convey only one idea or instruction at a time.
- Use short sentences with a subject and verb.
- Phrase sentences in positive terms.
- Avoid using pronouns such as she, he, they, and it. Instead, refer to every object or person by name.
- Be patient and allow enough time for the person to hear and think about what you are saying.
- If necessary, repeat statements in the same way several times until you get a response.
- Use gestures or pictures to help get your point across.
- Never, under any circumstances, scold or reprimand the person.

Providing a Healthy Diet

Mealtime during the middle stage of Alzheimer's disease requires continuous supervision and assistance from the caregiver. You may have to cut your loved one's food into bite-size pieces. Take special care when serving hot foods because the person may no longer be able to feel the sensation of heat or respond to it. It is safer to serve food moderately warm. The person may hold food in his or her cheeks and not swallow regularly. If this happens, the caregiver should remind the person to swallow or periodically check inside the person's mouth. If food is present, gently knead his or her cheeks. In some cases, the person may hide food, spit food out, or try to eat nonfood items. Be prepared for these possibilities. If your loved one spits food out, try pureeing his or her food to ensure consistent textures.

It is a good idea to serve one course at a time, and provide only one utensil for each course. The dinner table or tray should be as uncluttered as possible; this will help the person focus on eating. Also, calm surroundings during mealtime will help to ensure that the person eats as much of the meal as possible.

Let your loved one feed himself or herself as much of the meal as possible and assist only when necessary. It is important to note that a person with Alzheimer's disease is usually able to feed himself or herself well into the middle stage of the disease. Once you begin feeding your loved one, he or she will begin to lose those skills, and you will probably have to feed him or her from that point on. Therefore, it is to everyone's advantage to postpone feeding the person until it becomes absolutely necessary.

If your loved one paces a lot, he or she probably needs to take in additional calories. Try giving him or her finger foods that he or she can hold in his or her hand and eat while pacing. Foods such as sandwiches, pretzels, carrots, apple slices, bananas, seedless grapes, crackers, and cheese strips are possible choices. If the person holds food in his or her cheeks, remind him or her to swallow.

Hygiene

Encourage the person to do as much of his or her personal grooming as possible. Give simple instructions, one at a time. Do not give a new instruction until he or she has accomplished the previous one. Do whatever you can to keep bath time as stress free as possible. Never begin a bath when the person is tired or hungry. Allow sufficient time for bathing, and let the person do as much for himself or herself as possible. Remember that the longer the person uses his or her skills, the longer he or she will maintain function.

People with Alzheimer's disease are often afraid of bathing, and of removing their clothing and being naked in front of another person. They often resist taking a bath or shower. If your loved one resists the idea of bathing, try some practical strategies. For example, let the person choose (within reason) when he or she wants a bath. Offer a couple of choices, such as now or half an hour from now. You may also want to switch to sponge baths at this point or use a bath bench so that the person does not have to sit down in the tub. Washing one part of the body at a time may also help prevent resistance or embarrassment. Fill the bathtub before bringing your loved one into the bathroom; the sound of running water can be frightening. Make sure that the temperatures of the water and the room are comfortable. Give him or her the washcloth and soap and provide simple bathing instructions. Wash his or her face and hair last, since water on the face and head can be upsetting. You may want to consider using dry shampoo if hair washing becomes too difficult to manage.

Dressing

A person with Alzheimer's disease may need help choosing his or her clothes and getting dressed. If possible, let the person choose between two outfits. He or she may need verbal instructions and some assistance getting into his or her clothing. Loose, comfortable clothing such as sweatshirts and sweatpants can make dressing (and undressing) easier for everyone.

Using the Toilet

During the middle stage of Alzheimer's disease a person should still be able to control his or her bowels and bladder but may need to be reminded to use the toilet. He or she may have trouble remembering where the toilet is and may sometimes end up urinating in a closet unless the bathroom door is clearly marked or left open. He or she may also need to wear absorbent disposable briefs (never refer to them as diapers) in case of accidents. And make sure that the person wears clothing that is easy for him or her to remove. It may be helpful to keep a commode near his or her bedside. Avoid placing items nearby that may be mistaken for a toilet, such as a wastebasket.

Behavior Problems

Behavior problems most often occur during the middle stage of the disease. Anxiety and agitation are the most common behavior problems experienced by people with Alzheimer's disease. Following these basic guidelines will help you deal with these problems:

- Avoid getting into a power struggle with the person.
- Do not argue with the person.
- Do not confront him or her about memory loss.
- Do not scold the person for soiling himself or herself.

- Do not assume that his or her behavior is deliberate.
- Do not allow the person to become fatigued.
- Do not talk about the person with others when he or she is present.
- Maintain a peaceful, soothing environment.

Taking care of someone with Alzheimer's disease is a continual challenge. Try to get some assistance with caregiving during this stage so that you can rest, restore your strength, and maintain your objectivity and sense of humor. Contact a home healthcare agency that provides homemakers, companions, and home health aides to help people in your situation. For helpful advice on taking care of yourself, see chapter 13. Also see chapter 4 for information about choosing a home healthcare provider.

Late-Stage Alzheimer's Disease

A person with late-stage Alzheimer's disease needs total care. He or she will need to be bathed, dressed, and groomed and, because of incontinence, will need to wear absorbent disposable briefs at all times. During this stage of the disease, a person usually loses the ability to communicate with others, and his or her vocabulary decreases to just a few words. He or she may be unable to recognize familiar faces or even his or her own reflection in a mirror. A person with late-stage Alzheimer's disease may have trouble walking, and it may appear to others that he or she will fall at any moment. However, allow your loved one to walk (with assistance, if necessary) as long as possible before confining him or her to a wheelchair.

Eating and Choking

A person with late-stage Alzheimer's disease may have trouble swallowing, making choking a real possibility. If the person begins to cough every time he or she eats, he or she may have swallowing problems. Giving pureed foods in small bites will help prevent choking. Always allow sufficient time for the person to chew and swallow each bite. Some people with late-stage Alzheimer's disease may have to be fed, while others may still be able to feed themselves, using utensils or their fingers. In any case, it is a good idea to let the person eat as much as possible on his or her own before beginning to feed him or her. If the person has a preference for sweet foods, you may be able to get him or her to eat the entrée by lightly coating it with something sweet such as applesauce.

The Heimlich Maneuver for Choking

All caregivers need to be familiar with the Heimlich maneuver so they can help if the person they are caring for is choking. The Heimlich maneuver is usually taught in cardiopulmonary resuscitation (CPR) courses sponsored by a local chapter of the American Heart Association or the American Red Cross. Caregivers should also learn to administer CPR. Check with your local hospital for information about CPR classes in your area.

If the person can speak, cough, or breathe, then he or she is moving air through the airway. Do not interfere in any way with his or her efforts to cough out a swallowed or partially swallowed object.

If the person cannot breathe:

STEP 1.   Move the person to a standing position.

STEP 2.   From behind the person, place your fist with the thumb side against his or her stomach slightly above the navel and below the ribs and breastbone. Be careful not to touch the breastbone.

STEP 3.   Hold your fist with your other hand and give several quick forceful upward thrusts. This will increase pressure in the abdomen, which pushes up the diaphragm. This, in turn, increases the air pressure in the lungs and will often force the object out of the windpipe. Do not squeeze on the person's ribs with your arms—use only your fist in the abdomen. It may be necessary to repeat the procedure 6 to 10 times.

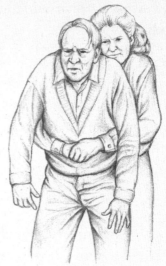

In some situations, you may not be able to move the choking person to a standing position. For example, he or she may be confined to bed or to a wheelchair. If the person is confined to a wheelchair, stand behind the chair and reach around the chair back and perform steps 2 and 3 on the previous page. If the person is bedridden, move him or her to a sitting position and perform steps 2 and 3 on the previous page from behind the person (while kneeling with one leg on the mattress if necessary). If you cannot move a bedridden person to a sitting position, turn him or her to one side, and reach around the person from above and beneath to perform steps 2 and 3 on the previous page. If the choking person is difficult to move, get another caregiver to help you immediately.

If the person is lying down:

STEP 1.   Turn the person on his or her back.

STEP 2.   Straddle the person, and put the heel of your hand on his or her stomach, slightly above the navel and below the ribs. Put your free hand on top of your

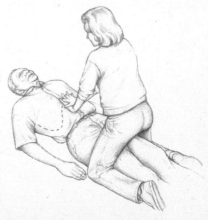

other hand to provide additional force. Keep your elbows straight.

STEP 3.   Give several quick, forceful downward and forward thrusts toward the person's head in an attempt to dislodge the object. Doing so will increase pressure in the abdomen, forcing pressure into the lungs to expel the object out of the windpipe and into the mouth. It may be necessary to repeat the procedure 6 to 10 times.

Dental Care

It is important to routinely observe the condition of a person's teeth and gums during late-stage Alzheimer's disease. Poorly fitting dentures and decayed teeth can lead to serious infections that can make this stage of the disease more difficult to manage. Swelling and bleeding of the gums are indications of gum disease. Sensitivity to hot and cold drinks may be a symptom of tooth decay. Watch carefully for these problems when feeding your loved one or when brushing his or her teeth. Talk to your dentist about the possibility of office visits or house calls. If your dentist does not have experience treating people with Alzheimer's disease, or if he or she is reluctant to do so, ask him or her for a referral. You might also check the yellow pages or contact the local dental association to find a dentist in your area who has experience treating people with Alzheimer's disease and who will make house calls, if necessary.

Communication and Interaction

Although a person with late-stage Alzheimer's disease may seem to be in his or her own world most of the time, it is still important to provide some type of stimulation during this stage of the disease. This can include talking or reading to the person, applying body lotion, giving back rubs, brushing his or her hair, and playing soft music. Although your loved one may not understand what you are saying or doing, he or she will respond to your demeanor, your touch, and the tone of your voice. These types of activities can enhance your loved one's quality of life.

Support Groups for the Caregiver

Being a caregiver for a person with Alzheimer's disease is both physically and emotionally challenging and can take a toll on your health. Taking care of your own needs first and accepting offers of help from other people will enable you to be a better caregiver. This topic is discussed in detail in chapter 13, but you should know that the Alzheimer's Association has hundreds of support groups throughout the United States for caregivers and family members. These support groups are open to anyone who is interested in attending and usually meet at least once a month. A support group may be of help to you and other members of your family by providing comfort and a place where you can openly express your feelings and share experiences with other caregivers. Support groups are a good source of helpful information and advice. Call the Alzheimer's Association at (800) 272-3900 to locate a support group in your area.

12

Caring for a Person Who Is Terminally Ill

Although it is a difficult emotional and physical challenge to care for a loved one who is dying, the experience can also be positive if you know what to expect and what to do. When there is no hope of recovery and death is inevitable, the caregiver's goal is to do everything possible to help the person die peacefully, with dignity and without pain. The process of dying is different for each person. The process may be relatively brief for a person with a progressive illness such as cancer, or it may occur gradually over the course of a number of years with a disease such as Alzheimer's.

Advance Directives

At some point, a person who is terminally ill may become unable to make decisions about his or her medical treatment. When this occurs, healthcare decisions are usually made by a close family member and the person's doctor. Advance directives are legal documents that provide guidance and instructions to ensure that any healthcare decisions that are made on a person's behalf are consistent with his or her wishes. Advance directives may be general statements about a person's attitudes toward heroic lifesaving measures and end-of-life medical treatment, or they may be detailed lists of the specific types of medical treatment a person does or does not want to receive. Living wills and durable power of attorney for healthcare are the most common types of advance directives.

Ideally, advance directives should be prepared and signed long before the need for them arises. The person can continue to make his or her own decisions about medical treatment as long as he or she is competent to do so. Advance directives go into effect when that is no longer possible and can be withdrawn at any time if the person changes his or her mind. If the person is able to do so, he or she should discuss the topic of advance directives with his or her physician, family, friends, and a member of the clergy. This will give the person an opportunity to sort out his or her feelings about life-sustaining medical treatments and make his or her wishes known to others.

Legal forms for advance directives are usually available through a hospital social services department or from local or state medical societies or bar associations. You can also get a form that was designed jointly by the American Medical Association, the American Bar Association, and the American Association of Retired Persons (AARP) by contacting AARP directly (see page 223). Also, a lawyer can work with you to create a living will and durable power of attorney for healthcare that suits the particular needs of your loved one. Although it is not necessary, it is a good idea to consult an attorney when preparing or filling out forms for a living will or durable power of attorney, because laws and requirements regarding advance directives vary from state to state.

Your loved one's doctor and close family members or friends should be told about these advance directives. The doctor and the person who has been chosen to make healthcare decisions on behalf of your loved one should receive copies of the directives. If healthcare institutions are involved, they should also receive copies so that they are aware of the person's wishes regarding medical treatment. The person should also keep his or her own copy where it can be located easily. Review these documents regularly and keep them up-to-date.

Durable Power of Attorney

A durable power of attorney is a legal document in which a competent person gives another person (called a proxy) the authority to make legal and financial decisions on his or her behalf. The proxy may be a relative, friend, lawyer, or guardian. The person may also name a second and third alternate proxy. A durable power of attorney goes into effect as soon as it is signed. It is not a substitute for a will and is effective only as long as the person is alive; the proxy has no power to make legal or financial decisions after the person has died. Also, the person can withdraw the power of attorney at any time.

Durable Power of Attorney for Healthcare

A durable power of attorney for healthcare is similar to the document described above, but it covers healthcare decisions only. A durable power of attorney for healthcare goes into effect only after the person is no longer competent to make his or her own medical decisions. The healthcare proxy is usually a close family member or friend, but in some cases may be the person's lawyer or guardian. A durable power of attorney for healthcare may also name a second and third alternate proxy. The healthcare proxy has the right to access medical records, consent to or refuse treatment, and withdraw life-sustaining treatment. The healthcare proxy also has the authority to make anatomical gifts, or organ donations. The proxy is expected to exercise good judgment and act according to the person's wishes. The person can withdraw the durable power of attorney for healthcare at any time.

Living Wills

A living will is a legal document that contains written instructions for medical personnel and loved ones regarding a person's wishes about medical treatment. A living will may be written in general terms or it may be specific. For example, it may state simply that the person does not want any extraordinary measures taken to prolong his or her life when he or she is terminally ill, or it may list the types of life-sustaining medical treatments he or she does or does not want to receive. These treatments can include measures such as cardiopulmonary resuscitation (CPR), artificial breathing with a ventilator, artificial feeding through a tube, a blood transfusion, and chemotherapy.

A living will is prepared when a person is still able to make his or her own decisions about healthcare; it is activated when the person can no longer make or communicate his or her choices about treatment and is considered terminally ill by his or her physician. A living will may be changed or withdrawn by the person whenever he or she chooses to do so. The requirements for and legal authority of living wills vary from state to state; a living will that is legally binding in one state may not be binding in another. Therefore, it is a good idea to consult a lawyer when preparing a living will.

Do-Not-Resuscitate Orders

A do-not-resuscitate (DNR) order is a legal directive stating that no one should perform CPR or take any other steps to revive a person if his or her heart stops beating. A DNR order is prepared and issued by a physician after discussing the matter with the person who is ill and his or her family members (or healthcare proxy). If it is an advance directive, both the person and his or her physician sign the order. However, if the person is no longer competent, a family member or healthcare proxy signs the order instead. In a hospital setting, only the person's physician signs the order. A DNR order can be withdrawn at any time.

Copies of the physician's written DNR orders should be kept in the person's medical record, whether the record is in a hospital, nursing facility, or home healthcare agency. If there are no written DNR orders signed by a physician, all medical personnel are required to begin CPR if the person's heart stops beating. If cardiac arrest occurs in a hospital setting, the person is usually attached to a ventilator for artificial breathing. Because these measures to revive a person may be in direct contradiction to his or her wishes or those of the family, it is important to discuss this issue long before a problem occurs.

Hospice

Hospice is a special type of care provided for people who are terminally ill and whose life expectancy is determined by a doctor to be 6 months or less. The purpose of hospice care is to allow a person to die with dignity in a comforting atmosphere, with minimal pain, and surrounded by close family members and friends. Hospice care is usually given in the person's home, but may be provided in a hospital, nursing home, or a hospice residence. The hospice care team usually includes a doctor, nurse, social worker, home health aide, clergy member, volunteers, and family members. Anyone whom the dying person regards as a family member, including close friends and same-sex partners, is regarded and treated as such by the rest of the team members. The primary caregiver is usually a spouse, partner, family member, or close friend. Other members of the hospice care team make regular visits to provide care, companionship, and support.

The hospice philosophy views death as a normal part of life. Hospice care does not interfere with the natural process of dying. Rather, it emphasizes quality of life by providing comfort and support for the dying person and his or her loved ones. Hospice care team members work together to provide day-to-day care, control of symptoms, pain relief, and emotional support. It is important to understand that home care is not provided on a 24-hour basis, but hospice staff is on call 24 hours a day, 7 days a week, should any problems arise. Hospice staff is trained to deal with all of the emotional issues associated with dying and death. Bereavement counseling for the person's family members and friends may be provided for up to 1 year after his or her death.

Services available through hospice programs usually include physician services, nursing services (including home health aides), medications (for pain relief and symptom control), respiratory therapy, medical equipment and supplies, and short-term hospitalization. Some programs may also provide homemaker services, social services, and counseling (including spiritual and bereavement counseling). Hospice care is usually provided based on need rather than on a person's ability to pay. Some hospice programs receive part of their funding through grants and donations. Medicare and most private insurers pay for the cost of hospice care. In addition, Medicaid programs in many states and some health maintenance organizations and other managed care plans cover the cost of hospice care. Hospice care may also be paid for out of pocket. If you are interested in a specific program, be sure to find out in advance about its payment policies and contact your loved one's insurer to determine if it covers hospice care. When choosing a hospice program for a person on Medicare, make sure that the program is certified by Medicare.

If possible, it is a good idea to discuss the possibility of hospice care with your loved one before the need for such care arises. Ask your physician or hospital social worker for a referral to a hospice program if you think that this type of care may be appropriate for your loved one and for you. Contact the National Hospice and Palliative Care Organization at (800) 658-8898 to request additional information and a complete list of hospice organizations in your area.

Relief of Symptoms

Many symptoms that occur during a terminal illness can be relieved, controlled, or eliminated. The following sections describe what you, the caregiver, can do to help the person and provide comfort.

Constipation

Constipation is a common symptom of a terminal illness. It can be relieved by giving the person foods that are high in bulk and fiber, such as prune juice and bran cereal, and making sure that he or she drinks a sufficient amount of fluids. Give stool softeners and laxatives as the doctor recommends. Constipation is also a common side effect of some pain medications and can be prevented by using stool softeners. For severe constipation, the doctor may prescribe a stronger medication. In general, the person should have a bowel movement at least once every 3 days. If he or she does not have a bowel movement after 3 days, notify the doctor or the hospice nurse as soon as possible.

Eating and Drinking Problems

Problems with eating and drinking are common in people with a terminal illness. You can help the person eat better by providing small, frequent meals. Cut food into bite-size pieces and serve it on a small plate. Depending on whether the person can tolerate it, some physical activity, such as sitting up in bed, getting out of bed and walking around, or range-of-motion exercises (see page 114) may help stimulate the appetite and aid digestion. Ask the doctor if the person should drink a liquid dietary supplement.

Dehydration can occur rapidly in people who are not drinking enough fluids. To prevent dehydration, have the person sip small quantities of fluids through a straw, or, if he or she is unable to tolerate fluids, offer ice chips to suck. Avoid overloading the person with fluids. Also, giving intravenous fluids to a person who is dying can result in respiratory distress. Carefully follow your doctor's instructions about providing food and fluids to your loved one.

Breathing Problems

Breathing problems can occur during the final stage of any illness and may require the use of oxygen. If oxygen is present in the home, never allow anyone to smoke. Raising the head of a person's bed or having him or her sleep in a recliner may help relieve breathing problems. Small doses of liquid morphine or bronchodilator drugs (available only with a doctor's prescription) may also help. Running a fan in the person's room can help improve air circulation.

Nausea and Vomiting

Nausea and vomiting may occur during a terminal illness, either as a side effect of medication or as a result of the disease itself.

Never force the person to eat if he or she is feeling nauseated. Antiemetic drugs (drugs used to prevent vomiting) may be helpful. If the person is vomiting frequently and cannot keep anything down, including medication, you may need to give the drug in suppository form.

Hiccups

Hiccups are sudden, involuntary contractions of the diaphragm (the sheet of muscle that separates the chest from the abdomen) followed by rapid closing of the vocal cords. Sipping water slowly through a straw can usually relieve hiccups. In some cases, however, if attacks of hiccups are frequent or persistent, the person may need to take medication to relieve them.

Dry Mouth

Dry mouth can be caused by medication or by the disease itself. You can help alleviate this problem by offering the person frequent sips of ice water or by having him or her suck on hard candies. You can use lemon glycerin swabs to wipe the inside of his or her mouth and the teeth. Use a light coating of petroleum jelly or lip balm to relieve dry, cracked lips. Artificial saliva is a mouth moisturizer that you can use to relieve dry mouth; ask the physician for a prescription.

Itching

Itching may have a number of causes, including dry skin, harsh soap, or laundry product residue in clothing and bed linens. To stop the itching, apply a soothing (alcohol-free) skin cream or calamine lotion liberally to the itchy areas, or try gently rubbing the skin with cornstarch, baking soda, or baby powder. Do not use skin creams or lotions that contain alcohol, because they will make the skin even drier. Using a humidifier during the fall and winter when the heat is on may help prevent or decrease the severity of dry skin.

Pain Control

Pain is a common problem with terminal illness. Pain control is the responsibility of the person's doctor and caregivers. Pain control enhances the quality of a person's life during the terminal phase of an illness. In the past, some doctors and families expressed concern that a dying person would become addicted to pain medication, an attitude that often resulted in inadequate pain relief and needless suffering. Today, however, most people realize that drug addiction is not a realistic concern at this time and they stress that keeping a terminally ill person as pain free as possible is the major goal.

Doctors often prescribe long-acting morphine to control the pain of a terminal illness, such as cancer. If pain recurs between doses, the doctor may also prescribe a shorter-acting form of the drug or another painkiller to use between doses of the longer-acting medication. In any case, it is important to give pain medication on a regular basis to ensure continuous pain relief; once pain begins to worsen, it is more difficult to control. To keep pain under control, experts usually recommend giving pain medication "around the clock," not just when a person asks for it. If pain medication has been prescribed on an "as needed" basis, the medication should be given as soon as the person begins to feel uncomfortable. Never wait until the person is experiencing pain before giving pain medication; doing so can cause him or her unnecessary suffering and distress. If the person is taking pain medication and is still in pain, talk to the doctor or the visiting nurse; it may be necessary to adjust the dosage.

Other pain-relief methods can be used along with medication to help control pain and improve the person's sense of well-being. These methods include relaxation techniques such as deep breathing, meditation, guided imagery, and massage. In general, the earlier a person begins to use relaxation techniques and massage for pain relief, the more likely these methods are to be effective.

Relaxation Techniques

Relaxation techniques help not only to relieve pain, but they can also help reduce the feelings of anxiety, anger, and depression that often accompany terminal illness. However, remember that relaxation techniques are to be used as a complement to and never as a substitute for pain medication. A dying person should never be allowed or encouraged to endure pain for any reason.

A combination of deep breathing, meditation, and guided imagery exercises is often an effective way to produce a state of complete relaxation. Give your loved one the following step-by-step instructions to slowly guide him or her through this exercise:

- Sit or lie in a comfortable position with your eyes closed.
- Relax all of your muscles.
- Inhale slowly and deeply.
- Exhale slowly and completely.
- Listen to each breath and try to concentrate on the rhythm of your breathing.
- Concentrate on a different part of your body for a few minutes as you breathe and relax. For example, tell the person to relax his or her face, neck, shoulders, right arm, left arm, right wrist, left wrist, right leg, left leg, right foot, and left foot.
- If your mind starts to wander, go back and focus on another part of your body.
- Finish up with a slow, deep breath as your entire body relaxes.
- Stay quiet for several minutes and slowly open your eyes.

You can help the person reach a state of total relaxation by speaking in a calm, soothing voice and providing reassurance and encouragement throughout the exercise. As a substitute for picturing various parts of his or her body, you might tell the person to picture a quiet place or a place that holds some special meaning, and ask him or her to picture that place in great detail. The person can also focus on a single word (such as "love" or "peace"), repeating it over and over again in his or her mind as he or she breathes in and out. For best results, encourage the person to perform this exercise for at least 10 minutes every day. Doing the exercise twice a day is even more beneficial.

Listening to relaxing music or watching a favorite movie or video can be enjoyable distractions that help reduce a person's awareness of pain. Reading to the person or simply sitting down and talking with him or her can also help the person focus his or her mind on something other than the pain. Some terminally ill people find that praying brings them comfort and helps them cope with pain.

Touch

As a caregiver, you should be aware of the power of touch. Most people, including those who are terminally ill, want and need to be touched. Touching is instinctive for humans, a basic element of everyday interaction. A person who does not experience touch can quickly begin to feel isolated. A caregiver can use touch to provide comfort, to reduce pain, and to communicate. Some common forms of touching are holding hands, hugging, and massage.

Do not be surprised or offended, however, if your loved one objects to being touched at certain times, in certain ways, or by certain people. If he or she does not want to be hugged or does not want a massage, do not take it personally. Everyone has the right not to be touched (beyond routine touching that occurs during caregiving), and no one should have to submit to unnecessary, unwanted touching. If your loved one appears to be uncomfortable or objects to being touched, discuss it with him or her. Ask how he or she feels about being touched. Find out what he or she likes and dislikes, and make sure that all other caregivers are aware of his or her preferences.

Massage is a good way to improve circulation, relieve pain, release tension, relax muscles, and improve mobility. A trained healthcare professional, such as a nurse or a physical therapist, can teach you the basics of massage while you watch him or her give your loved one a massage. Observe closely and ask questions. Ask the instructor to watch as you practice the techniques that you have just learned. At the very least, you will be able to give your loved one a good back rub from time to time.

For a relaxing back rub, have your loved one lie facedown on the bed. Remove any clothing from his or her back and slowly and gently stroke, rub, and knead the back. Rubbing a small amount of baby oil or lotion on the back can help make the massage more soothing. When you're finished, be sure to gently dab off any excess oil or lotion with a soft towel. Replace the person's clothing and help him or her return to a comfortable position.

Foot washing is another good way to use touch to help improve your loved one's sense of well-being. Have him or her sit in a comfortable chair while soaking his or her feet in a dishpan or other suitable container filled with warm water. Before the water cools, gently wash his or her feet with mild soap and a soft washcloth. Rinse the feet thoroughly and gently pat them dry with a clean, soft towel. Massage the feet with a small amount of petroleum jelly, baby oil, or an alcohol-free cream or lotion. Be sure to blot off any excess oil or lotion. A clean pair of soft cotton socks will keep the person's feet warm and help hold in moisture. Sheepskin heel protectors will help prevent pressure sores.

⚠️ **WARNING:** Never massage the legs, especially the calves, of a person who is confined to bed, because massage can easily dislodge a blood clot that has developed in the leg. The clot could then travel through the bloodstream to the lungs, resulting in a pulmonary embolism (blockage of an artery that supplies blood to the lungs). Symptoms of a pulmonary embolism include sudden difficulty breathing, chest pain, rapid pulse, sweating, slight fever, productive cough (a cough that produces sputum), and possible blood in the sputum. This condition is a medical emergency. If you notice these symptoms, call 911 or your local emergency number or take the person to the nearest hospital emergency department immediately.

Measuring the Effectiveness of Pain Control

To control your loved one's pain adequately, you need to know how well the pain medication is working. A simple way to determine the effectiveness of pain-control medication is to ask a person to describe the severity of the pain on a scale of 0 to 10, with 0 representing no pain and 10 representing the worst pain he or she has ever experienced. Ask your loved one to describe the pain before you give him or her pain medication. Then, about an hour after he or she has taken the medication, ask him or her to describe the pain again. If your loved one does not feel significant improvement, contact his or her physician or visiting nurse as soon as possible. The doctor can adjust the dosage or prescribe supplemental medication to improve pain control.

It is important to note that pain control must continue without regard to a person's level of consciousness. A person who is in a coma cannot communicate, but he or she can still experience pain. If the person is no longer able to take pain medication orally, these drugs can be administered in other ways. For example, some pain medications can be given intravenously through a special pump that can be programmed by the doctor or nurse to release the medication at intervals. In some cases, pain medications can be given through a skin patch.

Pain medication in suppository form is also available for people who are unable to take medications orally. To insert a suppository into the rectum, put on a disposable glove, turn the person on his or her side with the upper leg bent, and push the suppository deep into the rectum with the middle finger of your gloved hand. Most suppositories are self-lubricating. Sometimes, a doctor will recommend using an oral pain medication temporarily as a suppository. These drugs can be inserted into the rectum with a gloved finger that has been lubricated with petroleum jelly for easier insertion.

Side Effects of Pain Medications

Be extremely cautious with opioid pain medications, such as codeine and morphine, because they can cause sedation (drowsiness) when first administered or when the dosage is increased. Sedation that occurs when the dosage is increased should last only a day or two. If drug-induced sedation is persistent, the physician may recommend withholding the next several doses of the medication and decreasing the overall dosage. Notify the nurse or doctor promptly if the person becomes sedated. Urinary retention is another initial side effect of opioid pain medications, especially in men. Notify the nurse or doctor promptly if the person has not passed urine in more than 8 hours.

Constipation often accompanies the administration of opioid pain medications and can be treated with a high-fiber diet, increased fluid intake, stool softeners, and laxatives. Occasionally, constipation may require an enema. Nausea and vomiting, another side effect of pain medications, can be treated with antiemetic drugs. See sections in this chapter on constipation (page 162) and nausea and vomiting (page 163).

The initial side effects of opioids can be followed by increasing lethargy and labored breathing; the person's breathing gets slower and slower, and could stop. This is a medical emergency. If the person's breathing becomes labored, call 911 or your local emergency number, or take him or her to the nearest hospital emergency department immediately. If your loved one is in hospice, however, emergency procedures are not implemented.

Anxiety and Agitation

Anxiety and agitation can arise during the time leading up to death. You may notice your loved one pulling at the bedclothes, being restless, having insomnia, groaning, and continually fidgeting. Providing reassurance during this time is helpful, but often the problem is a physical response that can't be alleviated by reassurance. In this case, the doctor may prescribe an antianxiety medication such as alprazolam or lorazepam to help reduce the anxiety and agitation.

Be aware that the cause of the anxiety may in part rest on some unresolved personal issues. In this case, you may want to ask a member of the clergy to come to the home for spiritual guidance and direction.

Dying and Death

The term "dying" refers to the process in which the body's systems are shutting down and preparing for death. One of the symptoms that may occur during this time is rapid breathing (over 30 breaths per minute), which may be intermingled with periods (up to 15 seconds) of no breathing. Your loved one's arms and legs may become cold and may have a blue-purple coloring. The underside of his or her body may become darker in color as the circulation slows and blood begins to pool. He or she may begin to spend more and more time sleeping during the course of the day and may become difficult to arouse. In addition, he or she may pick at the sheets, covers, or pajamas, and stop communicating with people. He or she may have an increase in the amount and thickness of secretions in the back of the throat, resulting in a rattlelike sound. This is caused by the decrease in fluid intake and increasing inability to cough up saliva. Swallowing may become difficult, and the person may begin to refuse to eat or drink. Breathing may become shallower, the pulse weaker, and output of urine decreased. The actual moment of death is often very peaceful.

During the time that a person is "actively dying," the caregiver, family members, and visitors can help by sitting close to the person, holding his or her hand, talking softly to him or her, and stroking his or her hair. Tell the person you love him or her very much. Caution visitors not to talk about the person in front of him or her; although the person appears to be nonresponsive, he or she can hear and probably understands what you are saying. It is difficult to estimate how long this process will be.

If the person feels chilled, keep him or her covered with blankets (do not use electric blankets because of the possibility of burns). Keep the room at a comfortable temperature, and do not raise the thermostat. Using a humidifier in the room will help moisten the person's oral secretions. If breathing becomes difficult, you can elevate the head of the bed either by putting pillows under the person's head or, if you are using a hospital bed, by raising the head of the bed. Repositioning your loved one on his or her side may also help relieve a breathing problem. If he or she can eat, give only soft foods to avoid choking. Do not force the person to consume food or fluids at this time. Place incontinence pads or disposable briefs beneath the person to keep him or her dry. Change them whenever they become soiled, because skin can break down in a very short time when it's wet.

If your loved one is no longer able to speak, communicate through the sense of touch. This sense usually remains intact and helps to transmit feelings readily. Stroking and holding the person while gently speaking to him or her will convey your love and compassion. As a caregiver, you are dealing with an enormous amount of stress in handling your own grief while reassuring your loved one. If the person has been very ill for a long time, you may also feel a sense of relief about his or her impending death. This is entirely natural and part of the process.

If your loved one is in a hospice program, you may want to call the hospice team at this point. The nurse will come and give you help and support at this difficult time. If the person dies before the hospice team arrives, do not call 911. If you are not part of a hospice program, you will want to call your doctor at this time for further assistance.

You will know when death occurs by the following signs: breathing and heartbeat stop; bowel and bladder control stop, resulting in soiling of the bed linens; the person is completely unresponsive; his or her jaw is relaxed and the mouth is slightly open; the eyelids are slightly open and the eyes are fixed on a certain spot. The physician may want you to call 911 or may want to have the person brought to the hospital to be declared dead. Most undertakers will take the body to a hospital when directed to do so by a physician.

13

Care for the Caregiver

Taking care of yourself is an essential part of good caregiving. Because successful caregiving requires an enormous amount of time and energy, caregivers need to remain physically and emotionally healthy. If you are caring for someone who is ill, aging, or disabled, do not attempt to do everything yourself; the full responsibility of caregiving should never fall on one person. A caregiver who is on call 24 hours a day will burn out quickly.

Every member of the household should be expected to participate or contribute in some way. Some household members may claim they are too sensitive or too squeamish to assist in direct personal care. There are many other ways to help that do not require any special caregiving skills, such as doing chores, running errands, preparing meals, making telephone calls, and providing company. Be sure to schedule regular breaks from your caregiving duties so that you do not become overtired and irritable. You do not need anyone's permission to have some fun or to have a life of your own. And if you need a break at an unscheduled time, don't hesitate to ask for help. Perhaps you can arrange to have a dependable relative or friend fill in for you occasionally.

One of the most important things a caregiver needs to do for himself or herself is to identify as many people as possible who can help. Check with friends and relatives first. If help from them is not available, contact community and volunteer organizations, as well as your doctor and local hospitals and health organizations. You might also consider hiring a professional caregiver through a licensed home-health agency, such as a visiting nurse association (see page 64). The purpose of these organizations is to supply the assistance, guidance, and training you need to provide the best care possible for your loved one.

Taking Care of Yourself

Taking care of yourself will enable you to continue providing quality care to your loved one. Here are some guidelines that will help you cope with the demands of caregiving:

- Set realistic goals and limits. Educate yourself about your loved one's condition so that you know what to expect, now and in the future. This will help you to adjust your care plan as time passes. It will also help you avoid frustration and disappointment. Decide under what conditions you will no longer be able to care for your loved one at home and begin planning for that possibility well in advance. For example, if your loved one has early-stage Alzheimer's disease, you may want to begin gathering information about nursing homes in your area. If your loved one has a terminal illness, find out about hospice programs.

- Learn all you can about caregiving and make learning an ongoing process. There are many sources of useful information, including libraries, hospitals, agencies, and associations. Check the Resources section of this book for some recommendations.

- Do not confuse doing with caring. Recognize that your loved one will benefit from remaining as independent as possible for as long as possible. Resist the urge to do everything for him or her, and encourage your loved one to participate in his or her daily care routine.

- Get plenty of rest every day. Every caregiver needs an adequate amount of uninterrupted sleep at some time during the day, every day. Most people need between 7 and 8 hours of sleep each day. If possible, try to sleep at the same time your loved one is sleeping, or sleep while another caregiver takes over the caregiving tasks. Taking short naps or simply sitting down and resting for a few minutes throughout the day will also help keep you feeling energized. Remember, however, that catnaps and short breaks are no substitute for a good night's sleep.

- Be sure to keep all of your own medical and dental appointments. It is important that you stay as healthy as possible. Arrange to have a dependable family member, friend, or neighbor stay with your loved one while you visit your doctor or dentist.

- Maintain a healthy diet so that you always have enough strength and energy to get through all of the day's activities. Eat lots of fruits, vegetables, and whole grains, and be sure you are getting a sufficient amount of calcium every day. It's a good idea to take a multivitamin supplement every day to help ensure that you are getting the nutrients your body needs.

- Choose a type of exercise you enjoy and try to exercise every day. For example, 30 minutes of brisk walking each day will tone your muscles and stimulate your circulation (it will also get you out of the house).

- Make sure that you have a life of your own. On a regular basis, take time away from caregiving to enjoy yourself and take care of personal business. Don't neglect your personal life. Continue to participate in the activities that you have always enjoyed, especially those that will help take your mind off your caregiving responsibilities, even if only for a few hours at a time. Take long walks, go bicycling, go out to lunch or dinner with friends, or go to a movie or play. Go shopping. Make an effort to maintain your usual activities and interests.

- Take advantage of respite care when you need a break. A responsible family member or friend may be able to take over your caregiving responsibilities for several hours each week. Adult day care programs are often available through senior citizen centers and community service organizations, either free of charge or for a modest fee. Also, some hospitals and nursing facilities provide respite care services for longer periods of time (from several days to several weeks) for a fee. Your doctor can probably recommend respite care services in your area.

- Keep a diary throughout your caregiving experience. Writing things down at the end of the day can help you organize your thoughts, express your feelings, and find solutions to problems.

- Try to stay in touch with your feelings and find positive ways to deal with them. It is common for caregivers to experience feelings of guilt, anger, resentment, or depression. Don't ignore these feelings. If you don't address them, they can interfere with the caregiving process and have harmful effects on your health. Discuss your feelings with family, friends, and other members of the caregiving team. Joining a support group of caregivers can help relieve your sense of isolation and help you find ways to cope with your feelings and solve your caregiving-related problems. Watch for symptoms of depression (see page 23) and get professional help as soon as possible if you feel you are depressed.

Asking for and Accepting Help from Others

Some caregivers may find it difficult to ask others for help, even when they are feeling frustrated and exhausted. Some may refuse help when it is offered. This happens for a number of reasons. For example, a caregiver may feel that asking others for help is an imposition or that needing help is an admission of failure or incompetence. In some cases, a caregiver may believe that no one can do the job as well as he or she can, or he or she may feel an especially strong sense of obligation to the sick person. In some cases, the person being cared for might try to put pressure on the caregiver not to leave him or her or try to make the caregiver feel guilty. Most caregivers are women, and family members may pressure them to fulfill certain traditional roles.

Be honest with yourself about what you can and cannot do. If you are feeling that the responsibility is overwhelming, you may have trouble focusing on one aspect of the job when someone asks you how he or she can help. To be better prepared to accept offers of help, it is a good idea to keep a list of all the things that need to be done. For example, ask friends or family to come over one evening so that you can go out. Ask them to go shopping for you. Ask them to accompany you to the doctor's office either with the person who is ill or with you when you need to go.

Getting a Good Night's Sleep

Lack of sleep can harm your health and interfere with your ability to perform as a caregiver. If you are having problems falling asleep at night, or if you cannot sleep soundly, try some of the following suggestions:

- Go to bed and get up at the same time every day; a sleep routine programs your biological clock.
- Avoid taking naps. Too much napping during the day may leave you wide awake at bedtime.
- Exercise regularly during the day; this may help you sleep better at night. But avoid becoming overtired, which can make it harder to fall asleep.
- Avoid vigorous exercise right before bedtime; the stimulation can keep you awake.
- Take a warm bath before bedtime to help you relax.
- Perform relaxation techniques such as deep breathing exercises (see page 166) at bedtime.
- Sleep in a bed, not on a couch or in a chair. Being comfortable is an important part of getting a good night's sleep.
- Do not go to bed feeling hungry or soon after eating a meal. A glass of warm milk at bedtime may help you fall asleep.
- Avoid stimulants such as caffeine or nicotine before bedtime. They can keep you awake.
- Avoid drinking alcohol late in the evening. It can disturb your sleep.
- If you cannot fall asleep, get out of bed and do some light reading or listen to some relaxing music until you feel sleepy. Avoid watching television because it may serve as a stimulant and keep you awake.

Trying to do it all yourself is counterproductive and may even be dangerous. Sharing your caregiving responsibilities with others whenever possible helps ensure the quality of the care, the continuity of care, the health and well-being of the sick person, and your own health and well-being. Get in the habit of asking for help as soon as you need it. Do not wait until a situation becomes unmanageable. And do not hesitate to accept help when it's offered.

If you cannot rely on friends, neighbors, or family members, ask your doctor for a referral to a visiting nurse association, which can send a nurse in to evaluate the situation and provide some needed help. Consider hiring a homemaker, home health aide, or companion to help with the day-to-day tasks. If family members cannot give their time, perhaps they can offer to pay for some of the help you need. Some hospitals and nursing homes have respite facilities where you can bring your loved one for a short time while you go away on a trip, make up the needed sleep you might have lost, or just stay home and enjoy the solitude. Inquire about the governmental services the person may be entitled to that could help you with required tasks. This might include Meals on Wheels, homemaker services, respite care, shopping services, case management, Medicar, or taxi service. If you are involved with a hospice program, you may be able to arrange to have a hospice volunteer come and stay with the person while you spend some time away from home.

Depending on the illness that your loved one has, you may want to attend a support group in your community. The American Self-Help Clearinghouse on the Internet (http://www. selfhelpgroups.org) can help you review each of the hundreds of support groups nationwide and provide information about how to form your own support group. Most support groups have newsletters that describe different caregiving approaches you can take. Various national organizations for specific illnesses provide support and valuable information about all aspects of the condition. Internet users will benefit by receiving additional information about specific diseases and by developing social contacts with persons who have similar diseases. This resource can be invaluable to individuals and caregivers who are confined to home. Be skeptical, though, about some of the information offered on the Internet. Unless it is part of the educational material published by a reputable national organization, you cannot necessarily rely on the scientific credibility of the information. If you do not have access to the Internet, ask your librarian to help you find organizations that may be helpful.

Protecting Your Back

It is easy to injure your back when moving, lifting, or transferring a person. If an unskilled person tries to move someone, it can result not only in pain and chronic problems for the caregiver but also in a fall for the person being moved. It is helpful to have a hospital bed in the home if you are going to care for a

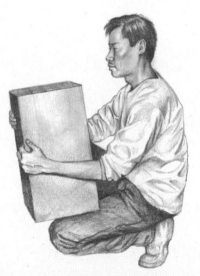

Proper Lifting
To help protect your back when you lift something off the floor, bend at your knees rather than at your waist, keeping your back straight and your head erect. Use the large muscles of the legs to raise yourself up again.

loved one for a period of time. Working with the bed at waist level will help prevent strains from leaning over. Install a trapeze over the person's hospital bed. This will enable the person to help lift himself or herself and make it easier for you to change pads, briefs, or sheets. If possible, get the person out of bed before you change the sheets; it is much more difficult to make a bed with the person in it. If the person remains in bed while you are making it, be sure to lower the bed to its lowest position after the linens are changed. If you need to change the linens with the person in the bed, see page 25 for helpful information.

Use a bath bench and handrails when giving your loved one a bath in the tub. This will help prevent you from straining to lift the person from the bathtub floor and enable the person to hold on to something when getting out of the tub. You may benefit by having a physical therapist from a home healthcare agency show you safe and effective ways to care for, move, and lift your loved one.

Stress Relief for Caregivers

Caring for a loved one at home can be a major cause of stress for the entire household, but it is especially stressful for the caregiver. The person you are caring for may be confused, angry, or depressed. He or she may be demanding or difficult to please, making you feel inadequate, frustrated, angry, and trapped. You may feel guilty for having these negative feelings.

Preventing Burnout

Burnout is physical or emotional exhaustion caused by, in this case, the prolonged stress of caregiving. For many caregivers, the natural tendency is to remain stoic, selfless, and constantly aware of their loved one's needs. But the costs of self-sacrifice can be high. Burnout can be debilitating, affecting your health and emotional well-being. Burnout also affects your ability to care for your loved one.

Burnout usually occurs gradually; the first signs and symptoms may not appear until long after the caregiver has settled into a daily caregiving routine. Because different people have different coping abilities, burnout levels vary from person to person. Some common signs of caregiver burnout include:

- Anger
- Irritability
- Feeling frustrated or overwhelmed
- Lack of energy; tiring easily
- Feeling isolated
- Crying regularly
- Difficulty handling minor problems or making minor decisions
- Blaming the sick person
- Overreacting to minor problems
- Frequent headaches or colds
- A change in appetite
- Sleep problems
- Skin problems, such as acne or rashes
- Inability to concentrate
- Feeling anxious, depressed, or resentful
- Nervous habits (such as nail biting, chain-smoking, or overeating)
- Exhaustion

To help prevent burnout, have a dependable support system in place consisting of people you can talk to or visit on a regular basis to express your feelings and concerns. Many caregivers are relieved just by having someone to talk to. If nothing is done to reverse or relieve it, burnout can quickly lead to depression.

Therefore, if you have any symptoms of burnout, seek assistance from a social worker, physician, nurse, psychologist, or professional counselor as soon as possible. A visit with a member of the clergy may also help.

Some people may find it helpful to consider caregiving from a philosophical or spiritual perspective and try to find a deeper meaning beyond the day-to-day tasks. Try to think of what you are doing as a meaningful, rewarding experience rather than as simply a job or an obligation. The satisfaction and pleasure that you can get from providing care for another person can help keep you motivated and energized when you begin to feel tired or frustrated. While caregiving is not always a personal choice, it is a generous act.

Taking Care of Your Own Needs

If you are a caregiver, respite can take a variety of forms. It may be something simple, such as enjoying a hot bath at the end of the day or watching a favorite television show. It can be an organized program, such as adult day care or a respite care program. In a respite care program, the person you are caring for goes to a hospital or another healthcare facility for care or treatment, or a respite worker or volunteer comes to stay with your loved one at home, allowing you to get away or spend some time alone.

You should also maintain activities and relationships outside the home as much as possible. If you are employed outside the home, for example, try to keep your job if at all possible. At the same time, try to continue to participate in pleasurable activities such as a sports league, a book discussion group, a hobby club, or volunteer work. Exercising regularly is one of the most effective ways to relieve stress. Here are some other simple things you can do to relieve stress:

- Listen to relaxing music.
- Take a long, quiet walk.
- Go out to dinner with a friend.
- Swim at a local pool.
- See a movie.
- Read a favorite magazine or book.
- Work out at a health club.
- Get a massage.
- Laugh as often as possible.

At times, it may seem like too much effort to continue participating in such activities. Or you may feel guilty about leaving your loved one while you go for a break or have some fun. But remember that it is not a good idea to take on all the caregiving responsibilities. Accept offers of help from others, including family members, friends, respite workers, and volunteers.

Make an effort to maintain relationships with those who genuinely care for you and who will make an effort to understand and empathize with you. While no one can fully comprehend what you are going through, good friends can listen, care, and provide a different perspective. They can help keep you balanced in a world that has been turned upside down as a result of your loved one's illness.

Many people find comfort in sharing their experiences with others in support groups. In such groups, people can express their concerns about particular diseases and chronic illnesses, such as diabetes, cancer, or Alzheimer's disease. Consult your local telephone book or hospital for information about groups in your area. Your physician or other members of your health-care team may also be able to recommend a support group. The Internet is also a good place to look for a support group that will meet your needs. If you cannot find a support group in your area, consider starting your own.

What You Can Do to Help a Caregiver

As a friend or relative of a caregiver, you can do many things to help make his or her job easier. Although these actions are relatively simple, they can have a profound, positive impact on a caregiver's day-to-day life.

- Keep in touch. Call or visit the caregiver as frequently as you can. Caregivers often feel isolated, and it can be a great relief to talk with friends or relatives. Encourage the caregiver to participate in outside activities. Invite him or her out to dinner and a movie. Be prepared to provide some laughter, too.

- Offer to help. Ask the caregiver what he or she would like you to do. Because many caregivers are reluctant to ask for help, you may need to be persistent. Make it clear that you want to help. You may not have much time to offer, but every contribution you can make will be a great help to the caregiver. You might suggest performing tasks such as running errands, making telephone calls, shopping, or staying with the person while the caregiver goes out—whether for an hour, an afternoon, or a day.

- Be a good listener. It is important for caregivers to discuss their feelings and concerns. Let the caregiver know that you are available if he or she needs to talk. Be sure to provide lots of support and encouragement. And remember, hugging is good for everyone.

Resources

The following list of organizations provides important details for care-receivers and caregivers who are searching for information on topics such as adult day care, aging, Alzheimer's disease, caregiving, health insurance, hospice, assisted living housing, legal services, and Social Security benefits.

The list is divided into the following sections:

- Diseases and Conditions
- General Health Information
- Government Agencies
- Health Information Web Sites
- Home-Care Services and Hospice
- Long-term Care and Housing
- Mental Health
- Rehabilitation
- Self-help and Support
- Senior Advocacy
- Miscellaneous

Most of the groups listed below have toll-free (800 or 888) telephone numbers; some also have TDD (telecommunication device for the deaf) numbers for people who are hearing impaired and TTY (teletypewriter) numbers for people who are hearing or speech impaired. Many groups in this list also have Web sites. You may write, call, or visit a group's Web site for additional information and assistance.

Diseases and Conditions

Alzheimer's Association
919 North Michigan Avenue, Suite 1100
Chicago, IL 60611-1676
phone: (800) 272-3900 or (312) 335-8700
fax: (312) 335-1110
web site: http://www.alz.org

The Alzheimer's Association sponsors advocacy, research, and education programs and offers care, support services, and referrals through a network of local chapters. The association also sponsors national conferences, events, and programs (such as Safe Return, a nationwide identification program for locating lost or disoriented people and reuniting them with their families). The Alzheimer's Association publishes *Advances*, a quarterly newsletter for families affected by the disease, and *Research & Practice*, a newsletter for health professionals. The association's Benjamin B. Green-Field Library & Resource Center has a wide range of informational materials (including books, journals, videos, audiocassettes, and CD-ROMs) available for use on-site or through interlibrary loan.

Alzheimer's Disease Education and Referral Center
P.O. Box 8250
Silver Spring, MD 20907-8250
phone: (800) 438-4380
fax: (301) 495-3334
web site: http://www.alzheimers.org

The Alzheimer's Disease Education and Referral Center (ADEAR Center) is a service of the National Institute on Aging (NIA), which is part of the National Institutes of Health. The ADEAR Center answers questions about Alzheimer's disease, including questions about research findings and new treatments. The center also offers free publications and can provide information on and referrals to diagnosis and treatment centers, drug trials, and support groups.

American Cancer Society
1599 Clifton Road, NE
Atlanta, GA 30329-4251
phone: (800) ACS-2345 (227-2345) (Info-line) or
    (404) 320-3333 (national office)
fax: (512) 927-5791 (Austin, TX)
web site: http://www.cancer.org

The American Cancer Society provides a wide range of services to
people with cancer, their families and caregivers, and the general
public. The society offers a number of educational programs and
support groups, free pamphlets and brochures, transportation to
and from medical treatments, lodging assistance, and camps for
children who have or have had cancer. The society's *TLC Cata-
logue* offers medical information and special products for women
who have recently been diagnosed with breast cancer, breast cancer survivors, and women with treatment-related hair loss.

American College of Cardiology
Heart House
9111 Old Georgetown Road
Bethesda, MD 20814-1699
phone: (800) 253-4636 or (301) 897-5400
fax: (301) 897-9745
web site: http://www.acc.org

The American College of Cardiology (ACC) is an international
professional society of cardiovascular physicians and scientists.
Members have special knowledge and experience in treating heart
disorders. The college offers patient education materials and
referrals for people who need the services of board-certified
cardiologists.

American Diabetes Association
1701 North Beauregard Street
Alexandria, VA 22314
phone: (800) DIABETES (342-2383) or (703) 549-1500
web site: http://www.diabetes.org

The American Diabetes Association (ADA) fights diabetes
through education and research. Local chapters provide a wide

range of services, including diabetes education classes, year-round youth programs, counseling and support groups, advocacy services, and referral services. The ADA sponsors a special African American Program designed to increase diabetes awareness among African Americans. The program offers community-based activities such as Diabetes Sunday, Get Up and Move, and Healthy Eating; a newsletter called *In Touch;* a health and wellness magazine for people with diabetes, called *Diabetes Forecast;* and a bimonthly newsletter, *Diabetes Advisor,* which provides easy-to-understand information on self-care for people who are learning to live with diabetes. The ADA also publishes books, brochures, and pamphlets on every aspect of living with diabetes, and a comprehensive collection of cookbooks, meal-planning guides, and food-exchange lists. You may purchase ADA books at your local bookstore or directly from the ADA. Call the organization's toll-free information and referral line or write to "Customer Service" to request a free diabetes information packet.

American Heart Association

7272 Greenville Avenue
Dallas, TX 75231-4596
phone: (800) AHA-USA1 (242-8721) or (214) 373-6300
web site: http://www.americanheart.org

The American Heart Association (AHA) is a nonprofit volunteer agency that strives to reduce death and disability caused by cardiovascular disease, such as heart disease and stroke, through education, advocacy, and research. The AHA publishes informational materials on all aspects of cardiovascular disease. The AHA Web site offers helpful information on topics such as warning signs, risk assessment, prevention, treatment, and recovery, and provides links to other online sources of useful information. The association's Web site also has an easy-to-use A to Z reference guide to heart disease and stroke.

American Stroke Association

7272 Greenville Avenue
Dallas, TX 75231-4596
phone: (888) 4-STROKE (478-7653)
web site: http://www.strokeassociation.org

The American Stroke Association, a division of the American Heart Association, provides nationwide information and referrals for people who have had strokes, their families and caregivers, and the general public. The people who handle the calls at the American Stroke Association can answer questions about stroke, help locate local support groups, provide information about how to subscribe to *Stroke Connection* magazine, or simply offer the caller the opportunity to talk to someone who understands.

Arthritis Foundation
1330 West Peach Tree Street
Atlanta, GA 30309
phone: (800) 283-7800 or (404) 872-7100
web site: http://www.arthritis.org

The Arthritis Foundation is a nonprofit volunteer organization dedicated to improving the quality of life for people with arthritis. The foundation supports research and offers continuing education programs and publications for healthcare professionals. Local chapters provide information and referral services for people with arthritis and their families. They also offer educational programs including self-help courses, exercise programs, and support groups. The Arthritis Foundation has a large selection of helpful brochures, booklets, videos, and other resources available free of charge or for a modest fee. The foundation also publishes a bimonthly consumer magazine for members.

Asthma and Allergy Foundation of America
1233 20th Street, NW, Suite 402
Washington, DC 20036
phone: (800) 7-ASTHMA (727-8462) or (202) 466-7643
fax: (202) 466-8940
web site: http://www.aafa.org

The Asthma and Allergy Foundation of America (AAFA) is a nonprofit organization that works to control and to find a cure for asthma and allergic diseases. The AAFA serves the public through research, educational programs for patients and the public, direct individual and family support through local chapters and educational support groups, public awareness campaigns, and advocacy.

The organization produces several subscription newsletters, including *The Asthma and Allergy Advance*, a bimonthly patient education newsletter, *HealthLines SAY*, a bimonthly newsletter written by and for adolescents who have asthma and allergies, and *Asthma & Allergy Exchange*, a quarterly newsletter for healthcare professionals. AAFA offers a number of asthma education programs and a variety of educational materials such as books, games, and videos that can be ordered from the foundation at a discount to members. Contact AAFA for additional information or to request a list of available materials.

Brain Injury Association, Inc.

105 North Alfred Street
Alexandria, VA 22314
phone: (703) 236-6000
Family Helpline: (800) 444-6443
fax: (703) 236-6001
web site: http://www.biausa.org

The Brain Injury Association (BIA) helps people locate and develop community-based resources, supports medical research and legislation, and sponsors conferences and meetings. The BIA Family Helpline offers consumers helpful information on topics such as preventing, treating, and living with a brain injury, as well as factors related to rehabilitation. The BIA also sponsors interactive multimedia Brain Injury Resource Centers, which provide easy-to-understand information for families and more complex information for medical professionals. The information includes answers to questions about brain injury, a glossary of medical and technical terms, and descriptions of professionals who deal with brain injury and the services they offer. Also available are interviews with people who are at various stages of recovery from a brain injury, their family members, and healthcare professionals, and a list of educational and informational materials.

Cancer Information Service

phone: (800) 4-CANCER (800-422-6237) or
    (800) 332-8615 (TTY)
web site: http://cis.nci.nih.gov

The Cancer Information Service (CIS) is supported by the National Cancer Institute, the federal agency that coordinates the government's cancer research programs. The CIS answers questions about cancer and cancer-related issues and offers free literature and other resources. The CIS also provides information on the most recent clinical studies and experimental treatment programs.

Heart Information Service
Texas Heart Institute
P.O. Box 20345
Houston, TX 77225-0345
phone: (800) 292-2221 or (713) 794-6536
fax: (713) 791-3714
web site: http://www.tmc.edu/thi/

The Heart Information Service, a program of the Texas Heart Institute, is a national hot line for questions about the diagnosis, treatment, and prevention of cardiovascular disease. The service is available to the general public.

International Hearing Society
16880 Middlebelt Road, Suite 4
Livonia, MI 48154
phone: (800) 521-5247; ext 333 (Hearing Aid Helpline)
fax: (734) 522-0200
web site: http://www.hearingihs.org

The International Hearing Society (IHS) is a professional organization that sets professional standards and offers continuing education programs for hearing aid specialists. The Hearing Aid Helpline operators answer questions about hearing aids and hearing loss, handle consumer complaints about hearing aids, and provide referrals to qualified hearing aid specialists. The Hearing Aid Helpline operates between 10 A.M. and 4 P.M. (Eastern Standard Time) Monday through Friday. The IHS publishes the *Directory of National Hearing Aid Society Members* and other publications that deal with specific questions about hearing aids and hearing loss.

International Tremor Foundation
7046 West 105th Street
Overland Park, KS 66212-1803
phone: (913) 341-3880
fax: (913) 341-1296
web site: http://www.essentialtremor.org

The International Tremor Foundation is a nonprofit membership organization that provides information and referral services for people who have tremor disorders and their families. The foundation supports research on tremor disorders and publishes a quarterly newsletter for its members. The organization also offers a variety of publications on tremor disorders.

National Institute of Arthritis and Musculoskeletal and Skin Diseases Information Clearinghouse
National Institutes of Health
1 AMS Circle
Bethesda, MD 20892-3675
phone: (301) 495-4484 or (301) 565-2966 (TTY)
fax: (301) 718-6366 or NIAMS Fast Fax System: (301) 881-2731
web site: http://www.nih.gov/niams

The National Institute of Arthritis and Musculoskeletal and Skin Diseases Information Clearinghouse is part of the National Institute of Arthritis and Musculoskeletal and Skin Diseases (NIAMS), which is part of the National Institutes of Health, the US government's principal biomedical research agency. The NIAMS supports and conducts clinical research and provides up-to-date information for both consumers and health professionals about issues and products related to arthritis and diseases of the musculoskeletal system and skin. The group provides fact sheets, brochures, health statistics, and reports, as well as scientific research databases and other biomedical resources on the Internet.

National Association for Continence
P.O. Box 8310
Spartanburg, SC 29305-8310
phone: (800) BLADDER (252-3337) or (864) 579-7900
fax: (864) 579-7902
web site: http://www.nafc.org

The National Association for Continence (NAFC) is a nonprofit membership organization that works to improve the quality of life for people with incontinence. The NAFC conducts education, advocacy, service, and support programs and focuses on causes, prevention, diagnosis, treatment, and management alternatives. The organization publishes *Quality Care*, a quarterly newsletter, and *The Resource Guide—Products and Services for Incontinence*, a directory of products and manufacturers. The NAFC also provides helpful information on dealing with incontinence.

National Association of the Deaf
814 Thayer Avenue
Silver Springs, MD 20910-4500
phone: (301) 587-1788 or (301) 587-1789 (TTY)
fax: (301) 587-1791
web site: http://www.nad.org

The National Association of the Deaf (NAD) is a nonprofit advocacy organization that serves the needs of people who are deaf or hearing-impaired. The association answers questions from the general public and supports a variety of programs, including Youth Leadership Camp, Junior NAD, Interpreter and Sign Language Interpreter certification, and the Legal Defense Fund. The NAD also offers a variety of books and other informative publications about hearing loss and deafness.

National Center for Vision and Aging
The Lighthouse International
111 East 59th Street, 11th floor
New York, NY 10022-1202
phone: (800) 334-5497 (Information and Resource Service) or
    (212) 821-9713 (TTY) or (212) 821-9200
fax: (212) 821-9705
web site: http://www.lighthouse.org

The National Center for Vision and Aging (NCVA), a division of The Lighthouse, Inc., assists older people who have, or who are at risk of developing, impaired vision. The NCVA conducts research on age-related vision impairment and provides a continuing education program for professionals. The NCVA Information and

Resource Service offers consumers helpful information on a variety of topics, including eye diseases and conditions and assistive devices, and can refer callers to vision rehabilitation agencies, low-vision centers, and support groups. The NCVA also produces a wide variety of educational materials for consumers. The *Lighthouse Consumer Catalog* offers a number of useful products for people who have impaired vision.

National Clearinghouse for Alcohol and Drug Information
P.O. Box 2345
Rockville, MD 20847-2345
phone: (800) 729-6686 or (800) 487-4889 (TDD)
fax: (301) 468-6433
web site: http://www.health.org

The National Clearinghouse for Alcohol and Drug Information is the largest resource for current information and materials about substance abuse and treatment. Many of these materials, including fact sheets, brochures, pamphlets, posters, and videotapes, are free. The group has both English- and Spanish-speaking information specialists who can recommend appropriate publications. Prevention Online (PREVLINE) is an interactive Web site where you can search for information about specific drugs.

National Diabetes Information Clearinghouse
1 Information Way
Bethesda, MD 20892-3560
phone: (301) 654-3327
fax: (301) 907-8906
web site: http://www.niddk.nih.gov

The National Diabetes Information Clearinghouse (NDIC) is an information and referral service of the National Institute of Diabetes and Digestive and Kidney Diseases (NIDDK). NDIC's purpose is to increase knowledge and understanding about diabetes. NDIC responds to written requests from consumers for information and offers a variety of fact sheets, brochures, pamphlets, booklets, reports, and reprints on diabetes. The group also publishes a quarterly newsletter, *Diabetes Dateline*, and *The Diabetes Dictionary*, an illustrated glossary of more than 350 diabetes-related terms. Search for additional information about diabetes on the Combined Health Information Database (CHID), which you can access from the NDIC Web site.

National Digestive Diseases Information Clearinghouse
2 Information Way
Bethesda, MD 20892-3570
phone: (301) 654-3810
fax: (301) 907-8906
web site: http://www.niddk.nih.gov

The National Digestive Diseases Information Clearinghouse (NDDIC) is an information and referral service of the National Institute of Diabetes and Digestive and Kidney Diseases (NIDDK). NDDIC's purpose is to increase knowledge and understanding about digestive disorders—including pancreatitis, inflammatory bowel disease, hepatitis, ulcers, and gallstones. NDDIC responds to written requests for information and offers consumers a variety of fact sheets, brochures, pamphlets, booklets, reports, and reprints on digestive diseases. The group's newsletter, *DD Notes*, features news and information about digestive diseases. Search for additional information on digestive diseases on the Combined Health Information Database, which you can access from the NDDIC Web site.

National Heart, Lung, and Blood Institute
Information Center
P.O. Box 30105
Bethesda, MD 20824-0105
phone: (301) 592-8573
recorded heart health information: (800) 575-WELL (9355)
fax: (301) 592-8563
web site: http://www.nhlbi.nih.gov

The National Heart, Lung, and Blood Institute (NHLBI) plans, conducts, and supports a program of research and education concerning diseases of the heart, lungs, blood, and blood vessels; blood resources; and sleep disorders. The NHLBI Information Center seeks to improve public health by translating the results of medical research into practical information and advice for consumers. The information center serves as a clearinghouse for brochures, audiovisual materials, cookbooks, and many more helpful materials.

National Institute of Diabetes and Digestive and Kidney Diseases

National Institutes of Health
31 Center Drive, MSC-2560, Building 31, Room 9A-04
Bethesda, MD 20892-2560
phone: (301) 496-3583
fax: (301) 496-7422
web site: http://www.niddk.nih.gov

The National Institute of Diabetes and Digestive and Kidney Diseases (NIDDK) is part of the National Institutes of Health, the US government's principal biomedical research agency. NIDDK conducts research and administers the National Diabetes Education Program, the National Diabetes Information Clearinghouse, the National Digestive Diseases Information Clearinghouse, the National Kidney and Urologic Diseases Information Clearinghouse, and the Weight-Control Information Network. The NIDDK publishes a variety of free fact sheets, brochures, and pamphlets for consumers on topics such as diabetes, digestive diseases, kidney and urologic diseases, weight control, and nutrition.

National Institute of Neurologic Disorders and Stroke

Office of Communications and Public Liaison
31 Center Drive, MSC-2540, Room 8A-18
Bethesda, MD 20892-2540
phone: (301) 496-5751
fax: (301) 402-2186
web site: http://www.ninds.nih.gov

The National Institute of Neurologic Disorders and Stroke conducts and supports research on the causes, prevention, diagnosis, and treatment of stroke and other disorders of the brain and nervous system. The group offers consumer-oriented publications on a variety of topics.

**National Kidney and Urologic Diseases
Information Clearinghouse**
3 Information Way
Bethesda, MD 20892-3570
phone: (301) 654-4415
fax: (301) 907-8906
web site: http://www.niddk.nih.gov

The National Kidney and Urologic Diseases Information Clearinghouse (NKUDIC) is an information and referral service of the National Institute of Diabetes and Digestive and Kidney Diseases (NIDDK). NKUDIC is designed to increase the knowledge and understanding about kidney and urologic diseases—including end-stage renal disease, urinary stone disease, urinary incontinence, benign prostatic hyperplasia, interstitial cystitis, urinary tract infection, and polycystic kidney disease—among people who have these diseases, their families, healthcare professionals, and the general public. NKUDIC responds to written requests for information and offers consumers a variety of fact sheets, brochures, pamphlets, booklets, reports, and reprints on kidney and urologic diseases. NKUDIC publishes a newsletter called *KU Notes*. Search for additional information on diabetes and urologic diseases on the Combined Health Information Database (CHID), which you can access through the NKUDIC Web site.

National Kidney Foundation
30 East 33rd Street
New York, NY 10016
phone: (800) 622-9010 or (212) 889-2210
fax: (212) 689-9261
web site: http://www.kidney.org

The National Kidney Foundation publishes pamphlets on kidney disease and offers health screening, counseling, referrals, transportation, and other programs for people with kidney disease.

National Osteoporosis Foundation
1232 22nd Street, NW
Washington, DC 20037-1292
phone: (202) 223-2226

fax: (202) 223-2237
web site: http://www.nof.org

The National Osteoporosis Foundation (NOF) is a volunteer organization that works to increase awareness and knowledge of osteoporosis. NOF supports osteoporosis research and works to increase federal funding for such research. The organization publishes a variety of materials for consumers, including *Osteoporosis: A Woman's Guide*, and *An Older Person's Guide to Osteoporosis*. NOF also publishes a quarterly newsletter and provides referrals to local osteoporosis support groups.

National Parkinson Foundation, Inc.
1501 NW 9th Avenue
Miami, FL 33136-1494
phone: (800) 327-4545 or (305) 547-6666
fax: (305) 243-4403
web site: http://www.parkinson.org

The National Parkinson Foundation is dedicated to finding the cause of and cure for Parkinson's disease and related disorders through research. The foundation works to educate medical professionals, patients, their families and caregivers, and the general public about Parkinson's disease. The foundation distributes a wide variety of free informational literature and sponsors seminars and support groups throughout the United States for people with Parkinson's disease and their families and caregivers. The group helps new support groups form by providing them with technical assistance and helpful informational materials. The foundation also provides complete diagnostic services as well as physical, occupational, and speech therapy for patients, regardless of their ability to pay. Call the toll-free number listed above to request materials, physician referrals, and general information.

National Stroke Association
9707 East Easter Lane
Englewood, CO 80112-3747
phone: (800) STROKES (787-6537) or (303) 649-9299
fax: (303) 649-1328
web site: http://www.stroke.org

The National Stroke Association is a nonprofit volunteer organization dedicated to stroke education and research. The association provides information, referrals, and guidance for forming support groups for people who have had strokes and their families and caregivers. The association also serves as a clearinghouse for information on prevention, detection, and treatment of stroke, and offers information on aftercare centers and rehabilitation.

Osteoporosis and Related Bone Diseases Resource Center
1232 22nd Street, NW
Washington, DC 20037-1292
phone: (800) 624-BONE (2663) or (202) 223-0344 or
    (202) 466-4315 (TTY)
fax: (202) 293-2356
web site: http://www.osteo.org

The Osteoporosis and Related Bone Diseases National Resource Center is dedicated to prevention, early detection, and treatment of osteoporosis and related bone diseases, as well as developing strategies to cope with the conditions. The center provides patients, healthcare professionals, and the general public with information and access to other resources.

Parkinson's Disease Foundation
710 West 168th Street
New York, NY 10032-9982
phone: (800) 457-6676
fax: (212) 923-4778
web site: http://www.pdf.org

The Parkinson's Disease Foundation is a nonprofit organization that provides a variety of services—including educational materials and programs, a quarterly newsletter, and physician referrals—to people who have Parkinson's disease and their families. The foundation supports neurologic research and also offers consumers a variety of helpful publications, such as *One Step at a Time* and *The Exercise Program*.

United Ostomy Association, Inc.
19772 MacArthur Boulevard, Suite 200
Irvine, CA 92612-2405
phone: (800) 826-0826 or (949) 660-9262
web site: http://www.uoa.org

The United Ostomy Association, Inc. (UOA) is a volunteer organization dedicated to assisting people who have had or will have intestinal or urinary diversions. The organization has local chapters throughout the United States. UOA provides preoperative and postoperative visits and support; publications about ostomy and alternate procedures; a quarterly magazine; advocacy activities; national, state, and regional conferences; and liaison to other healthcare organizations.

Y-ME National Breast Cancer Organization
212 West Van Buren Street, 5th floor
Chicago, IL 60607-3908
National Breast Cancer Hotline (24 hours a day, 7 days a week):
   (800) 221-2141 (English) or (800) 986-9505 (Spanish)
fax: (312) 294-8597
web site: http://www.y-me.org

Y-ME National Breast Cancer Organization is committed to serving women with breast cancer and their families and friends. Y-ME offers a national hot line, a Web site, and nationwide referrals to mammogram facilities, comprehensive breast centers, and treatment and research hospitals. Y-ME provides support programs, monthly educational and support meetings, public education seminars, special programs on breast health awareness for high school senior girls, and in-service workshops for healthcare professionals. Y-ME also works at the state and federal levels for increased breast cancer research funding, access to quality treatment for all women, and nondiscriminatory legislation. Y-ME has a network of local chapters and support groups and offers publications such as a bimonthly newsletter, *Hotline;* a bilingual newsletter, *Noticias Latinas;* and a variety of booklets about breast health and breast cancer. Most information is available in both English and Spanish. Contact the Y-ME National Breast Cancer Hotline for further information and assistance.

General Health Information

American Dietetic Association
216 West Jackson Boulevard, 7th Floor
Chicago, IL 60606-6995
phone: (800) 366-1655 or (312) 899-0040
fax: (312) 899-1979
web site: http://www.eatright.org

The American Dietetic Association (ADA) promotes the science of nutrition and public education about food, nutrition, and health. You can talk to a registered dietitian or listen to informative recorded messages about nutrition and health by calling the ADA's toll-free number. The ADA also publishes informational materials on a wide variety of nutrition-related topics.

American Medical Association
515 North State Street
Chicago, IL 60610
phone: (312) 464-5000
web site: http://www.ama-assn.org

The American Medical Association (AMA) is the largest physician organization in the United States. The AMA serves physicians and their patients by promoting ethical, educational, and clinical standards for the medical profession. Research on various age-related medical topics is often published in the *Journal of the American Medical Association (JAMA)* and other scientific journals. The AMA also publishes health information and medical news for consumers and physicians. The AMA Web site is an excellent place for consumers to look for useful information about disease prevention and health. Information about physicians is accessible by medical specialty or by doctor's name under Physician Select: The Doctor Finder on the AMA Web site. Referrals to licensed physicians throughout the United States are provided by county medical societies.

Canadian Medical Association
1867 Alta Vista Drive
Ottawa, Ontario
K1G 3Y6
phone: (613) 731-9331
web site: http://www.cma.ca

The Canadian Medical Association is a valuable source of medical information and resources. The group's Web site contains a search engine that helps locate links to a wide variety of medical topics.

National Health Information Center
P.O. Box 1133
Washington, DC 20013-1133
phone: (800) 336-4797 or (301) 565-4167
fax: (301) 984-4256 or (301) 468-1204
web site: http://nhic-nt.health.org

The National Health Information Center (NHIC) is a clearing-house that can help you find specific health organizations and information about the resources and services that they offer. If you do not know which organization to contact for specific health-related information, NHIC will direct you to the appropriate group.

National Medical Association
1012 10th Street, NW
Washington, DC 20001
phone: (202) 347-1895
fax: (202) 347-0722
web site: http://nmanet.org

The National Medical Association (NMA) is the collective voice of African American physicians and a leading force for parity and justice in the field of medicine and in healthcare. Consumers can visit the "Your Health" section of the NMA Web site to access up-to-date information on health issues such as breast cancer, glaucoma, AIDS, and asthma; to take action on legislative alerts; and to review the NMA calendar of events to find out about health-related events in their area.

Government Agencies

Consumer Product Safety Commission

Washington, DC 20207-0001
phone: (800) 638-2772 (English/Spanish) or
   (800) 638-8270 (TTY)
web site: http://www.cpsc.gov

The Consumer Product Safety Commission (CPSC) is an independent federal regulatory agency that develops and sets mandatory safety standards for manufacturers, educates the public about product safety, conducts research, and issues and enforces bans and recalls. The agency's purpose is to protect the public against unreasonable risks of injury and death associated with consumer products. The CPSC has jurisdiction over about 15,000 consumer products and operates the Injury Information Clearinghouse, which collects data about consumer product–related injuries. The agency also offers a variety of free publications, such as *Home Safety Checklist for Older Consumers* and *Fire Safety Checklist for Older Consumers*. Write to the agency to request a free copy of the CPSC publication list, or call for information about a specific product or to report an unsafe consumer product or a product-related injury or death.

Eldercare Locator

phone: (800) 677-1116

Eldercare Locator, a nationwide directory service established by the National Association of Area Agencies on Aging, provides state and local information and referrals for older people and their caregivers. Information and referrals are available for Alzheimer's disease hot lines, adult day care services, nursing home ombudsmen, home healthcare complaints, legal assistance, and elder abuse and protective services. Eldercare Locator answers calls Monday through Friday between 9 A.M. and 11 P.M. (Eastern Standard Time). After hours, voice mail will record your name and telephone number, and an information specialist will return your call the next business day.

Food and Drug Administration
5600 Fishers Lane
Rockville, MD 20857-0001
phone: (888) 463-6332 or (301) 827-4420 (in the Washington, DC area)
fax: (301) 443-9767
web site: http://www.fda.gov

The Food and Drug Administration (FDA) is the federal government's consumer protection agency. The FDA can provide information and answer questions about foods, food supplements, drugs, cosmetics, and medical devices—and how they are regulated.

Health Canada
AL 0904A
Ottawa, Ontario
K1A 0K9
phone: (613) 957-2991
fax: (613) 941-5366
web site: http://www.hc-sc.gc.ca

Health Canada is the government department responsible for helping Canadian citizens maintain their health. The department promotes disease prevention and healthy living. Health Canada's medical database provides helpful information on a variety of health-related topics.

National Institute on Adult Daycare
See National Council on the Aging, Inc., page 227.

National Institute on Aging Information Center
P.O. Box 8057
Gaithersburg, MD 20898-8057
phone: (800) 222-2225 or (800) 222-4225 (TDD, TTY)
fax: (301) 589-3014
web site: http://www.nih.gov/nia and http://www.aoa.dhhs.gov

The National Institute on Aging (NIA) is a branch of the National Institutes of Health, the principal biomedical research agency of the US government. The NIA promotes healthy aging by conducting and supporting biomedical, social, and behavioral research and public education. The NIA offers a wide variety of informative free brochures and fact sheets on topics of interest to older people. The literature, called *Age Pages*, covers topics such as specific diseases, health promotion and disease prevention, medical care, medications and immunizations, exercise, nutrition, planning for later years, and safety.

Office of Minority Health Resource Center
P.O. Box 37337
Washington, DC 20013-7337
phone: (800) 444-6472 or (301) 589-0951 (TDD)
fax: (301) 589-0884
web site: http://www.omhrc.gov

The Office of Minority Health Resource Center (OMH-RC) is a nationwide service of the Office of Minority Health (OMH). The OMH is part of the Public Health Service, US Department of Health and Human Services. The OMH is dedicated to promoting the health of American Indians and Alaskan Natives, African Americans, Asian and Pacific Islanders, and Hispanics. The OMH-RC answers requests for information about minority health concerns and provides referrals to appropriate organizations. Staff members can handle calls in both English and Spanish.

Social Security Administration
Office of Public Inquiries
6401 Security Boulevard
Baltimore, MD 21235-0001
phone: (800) 772-1213 or (800) 325-0778 (TDD and TTY)
web site: http://www.ssa.gov

For problems, information, or guidance about Social Security matters, first contact your local Social Security Administration office or call the toll-free number listed above. Phone lines (including TDD and TTY) are open from 7 A.M. through 7 P.M. Monday through Friday. The best times to call are mornings, evenings, at the end of the week, or toward the end of the month. If you have a touch-tone phone, recorded information and services are available 24 hours a day, including weekends and holidays. If you need additional help, write to the Social Security Administration at the address above. Social Security Online is the official Web site of the Social Security Administration. The Web site offers useful information and guidance about Social Security benefits and services.

Veterans Affairs, Department of
Office of Consumer Affairs (075)
810 Vermont, NW
Washington, DC 20420
phone: (800) 827-1000 or (202) 273-5771 (Consumer Affairs)
web site: http://www.va.gov

The Department of Veterans Affairs (VA) is the federal agency that oversees programs and provides benefits for military veterans and their dependents and beneficiaries. Benefits for eligible veterans include medical and dental care, vocational rehabilitation, and burial assistance. The publication *Federal Benefits for Veterans and Dependents* describes all the benefit programs and is available free from the VA.

Health Information Web Sites

CancerNet
web site: http://cancernet.nci.nih.gov

CancerNet is an online information service provided by the National Cancer Institute, the federal agency that coordinates the government's cancer research programs. CancerNet provides access to up-to-date, accurate information about cancer that is continually reviewed and revised by cancer experts. Available information includes fact sheets, publications, and news about cancer-related topics such as prevention, screening, detection, treatment, ongoing clinical trials, rehabilitation, and quality of life. CancerNet also provides access to PDQ, the National Cancer Institute's comprehensive cancer database, and links to other National Cancer Institute home pages and organizations that offer cancer information, support services, and other helpful resources.

Caregiving Online
web site: http://www.caregiving.com

Caregiving Online is an online support service from the monthly newsletter, *Caregiving* (see entry on page 212). This Web site provides an online support center, a caregivers discussion group, a caregiving journal, a gallery of poems and essays by family caregivers, and links to other Web sites that have valuable information and services for caregivers. Caregiving Online also provides access to hospice-related Web sites, which offer support and helpful information on caring for people who are terminally ill.

ElderNet
web site: http://www.eldernet.com

ElderNet is an online guide offering links to Web sites that deal with topics of interest to older people, including health, long-term care, legal assistance, financial planning, health and retirement benefits, specific diseases and conditions, alternative therapies, managed care, news, and entertainment. ElderNet's *Senior Lifestyles Directory* provides access to nationwide information about living options such as retirement communities, assisted living, home care, and nursing facilities.

HealthFinder
web site: http://www.healthfinder.gov

HealthFinder is a health information Web site for consumers developed by the US Department of Health and Human Services and other government agencies, and coordinated by the Office of Disease Prevention and Health Promotion. HealthFinder provides access to selected online publications, clearinghouses, databases, Web sites, support and self-help groups, government agencies, and nonprofit groups that produce reliable health-related information for consumers on a wide variety of health topics.

HeartInfo
web site: http://www.heartinfo.org

HeartInfo is an independent, educational Web site dedicated to providing information and services to people with a cardiovascular disorder. The site is geared toward consumers and offers information about heart disease, the latest news on treatment options, and products and services.

Information from Your Family Doctor
web site: http://www.familydoctor.org

Information from Your Family Doctor is a patient-education Web site published by the American Academy of Family Physicians (AAFP). The AAFP is a national, nonprofit medical association of family physicians, family practice residents, and medical students dedicated to promoting and maintaining high-quality standards for family doctors who provide continuing comprehensive health-care to the public. The information on the Web site is written and reviewed by physicians and patient education professionals at the AAFP, and is reviewed and updated on a regular basis. Consumers who visit this site can find useful information on hundreds of health topics of interest to people of all ages.

National Self-Help Clearinghouse
web site: http://www.selfhelpweb.org

The National Self-Help Clearinghouse provides information about and referrals to self-help groups nationwide. The clearinghouse offers technical assistance, advice, and training programs to established self-help groups, and also offers guidance to people who want to organize self-help groups. A list of clearinghouse publications is available.

NetWellness
web site: http://www.netwellness.org

NetWellness is an online consumer health information service that was developed by the University of Cincinnati Medical Center, Case Western Reserve University, and Ohio State University. NetWellness offers up-to-date, general information about medications, diseases and conditions, standard and alternative treatments, and general health and wellness. The confidential and anonymous "Ask an Expert" feature provides answers to specific health questions. NetWellness also provides links to other reliable, health-oriented Web sites.

Resource Directory for Older People
web site: http://www.aoa.dhhs.gov/aoa/resource.html

The Resource Directory for Older People is an online guide to a wide array of organizations that offer valuable information and services of interest to older people, their families and caregivers, healthcare and legal professionals, social service providers, librarians, researchers, and the general public. The directory, which lists names, addresses, telephone and fax numbers, e-mail addresses, and Web sites, is provided through the cooperative efforts of the National Institute on Aging and the Administration on Aging, both of which are part of the US Department of Health and Human Services. The directory is continually updated.

RxList
web site: http://www.rxlist.com

RxList is an online directory of more than 4,000 brand-name and generic drugs. The directory includes drugs that are currently available in the United States or are close to receiving approval from the Food and Drug Administration (FDA). You can search for information on a specific drug or a category of drugs. Each entry provides a description of the generic drug and a list of brand names under which the drug is marketed. Other useful information includes what the drug is used for, when the drug should not be taken, warnings, precautions, other drugs or substances that can interfere with the drug's intended effects, side effects, dosage, and estimated cost of therapy. RxList also includes a list of the 200 most frequently prescribed drugs (for 1995 to 1999) based on data from prescriptions filled in the United States.

SeniorNet
121 Second Street, 7th floor
San Francisco, CA 94105
phone: (415) 495-4990
fax: (415) 495-3999
web site: http://www.seniornet.org

SeniorNet is a nonprofit educational organization that teaches people over 50 to use computers and the Internet. SeniorNet Learning Centers throughout the United States offer a variety of classes for both beginners and people who are more experienced with computers. Members are offered discounts on computer hardware, software, and other materials. Members also have access to SeniorNet Online, a nationwide computer network. SeniorNet publishes a newsletter, *Newsline*, and a variety of pamphlets on computer-related topics.

Third Age
web site: http://www.thirdage.com

Third Age is a Web site that provides access to a wide range of information, services, and other resources of interest to active older people. Topics include healthy living, caregiving, retirement housing, family, and financial management. Third Age also offers chat rooms and forums where older adults can express their views and share advice and experiences with others. Visitors to this Web site will also find online features such as a bookstore, news, and entertainment.

Home-Care Services and Hospice

Caregiving
Tad Publishing Company
P.O. Box 224
Park Ridge, IL 60068
phone: (847) 823-0639

Caregiving is a monthly newsletter that provides advice and support to people who are caring for an aging relative, friend, or neighbor. Caregivers will find valuable information on topics such as community services, emotional issues, skin care, lifting techniques, purchasing home medical equipment, hiring home health-care aides, and self-care. Readers can submit questions to a team of home-care experts that includes two social workers, a home medical equipment supplier, a Medicare billing specialist, and dementia care specialists. Subscribers also have the opportunity to purchase products and services at a discount through the Caregivers Club.

Meals on Wheels Association of America
1414 Prince Street, Suite 302
Alexandria, VA 22314
phone: (703) 548-5558
fax: (703) 548-8024
web site: http://mowaa.org

Meals on Wheels programs deliver nutritious meals to people who are unable to leave home or to prepare meals for themselves. Call the Meals on Wheels Association of America number for additional information.

National Alliance for Caregiving
4720 Montgomery Lane
Bethesda, MD 20814
phone: (301) 718-8444
fax: (301) 652-7711

The National Alliance for Caregiving provides information and referrals to national organizations that can help caregivers.

National Association for Home Care
228 Seventh Street, SE
Washington, DC 20003
phone: (202) 547-7424
fax: (202) 547-3540
web site: http://www.nahc.org

The National Association for Home Care (NAHC) is a trade organization that serves home care agencies, hospices, and home health aide organizations. The NAHC develops professional standards for home care agencies, provides continuing education programs for home health aides, and monitors federal and state legislation pertaining to home care and hospice. The NAHC provides listings of all local home care agencies, information on the types of services they offer, and material on selecting a home care agency. Consumers may access the Home Care/Hospice Agency Locator on the NAHC Web site to find home care providers in their area.

National Caregiving Foundation
801 North Pitt Street, Room 116
Alexandria, VA 22314
phone: (703) 299-9300
Caregiver Support Kit request line: (800) 930-1357
fax: (703) 299-9304

The National Caregiving Foundation offers free information for caregivers of people who have Alzheimer's disease.

**National Hospice and Palliative
Care Organization**
1700 Diagonal Road, Suite 300
Alexandria, VA 22314
phone: (800) 658-8898 or (703) 243-5900
web site: http://www.nhpco.org

The National Hospice and Palliative Care Organization (NHPCO) is a private, nonprofit group dedicated to promoting and maintaining compassionate, quality care for people who are terminally ill and their families. The group also works to educate the general public and health professionals about hospice and to make hospice care an integral part of the US healthcare system. The NHPCO publishes *The Guide to the Nation's Hospices*, a comprehensive listing of hospices throughout the United States. Consumers may call the NHPCO's toll-free number for referrals to local hospice programs. The NHPCO also maintains a comprehensive library of materials on hospice care (including books, directories, audiotapes, and videotapes). Various publications and hospice-related products are available for sale through the NHPCO store.

Visiting Nurse Associations of America
11 Beacon Street, Suite 910
Boston, MA 02108
phone: (617) 523-4042
fax: (617) 227-4843
web site: http://www.vnaa.org/home.htm

The Visiting Nurse Associations of America (VNAA) is the official national association of freestanding, not-for-profit, community-based visiting nurse agencies (VNAs). The VNAA provides effective, innovative, and personalized community-based home healthcare. Through its Web site, the VNAA offers advice on choosing a visiting nurse agency and provides answers to commonly asked questions about home care. The VNAA Referral System can help you locate a visiting nurse agency in your area.

Long-term Care and Housing

American Association of Homes and Services for the Aging
901 E Street, NW, Suite 500
Washington, DC 20004-2011
phone: (202) 783-2242
fax: (202) 783-2255
web site: http://www.aahsa.org

The American Association of Homes and Services for the Aging (AAHSA) is a trade association that represents over 5,000 non-profit nursing facilities, continuing care retirement communities, senior housing facilities, and community service providers. The AAHSA provides consumer-oriented information on long-term care and housing options such as nursing homes, continuing care retirement communities, and assisted living facilities. This information can help you to determine your needs, and then locate and evaluate accredited facilities and services.

Assisted Living Federation of America
10300 Eaton Place, Suite 400
Fairfax, VA 22030
phone: (703) 691-8100
fax: (703) 691-8106
web site: http://www.alfa.org

The Assisted Living Federation of America (ALFA) is a trade association devoted to promoting the interests of assisted living providers (assisted living facilities and related organizations) and enhancing the quality of life of people who reside in assisted living facilities. The group offers a list of assisted living residences by state and a free consumer brochure and checklist that contains information on how to choose and evaluate these facilities.

National Citizens' Coalition for Nursing Home Reform
1424 16th Street, NW, Suite 202
Washington, DC 20036-2211
phone: (202) 332-2275
fax: (202) 332-2949
web site: http://www.nccnhr.org

The National Citizens' Coalition for Nursing Home Reform is a nationwide consumer-advocacy group that works to ensure the quality of long-term care services. The coalition achieves its goals through consumer information and education, advocacy, citizen action groups, ombudsman programs, and enforcement of consumer-directed health, living, and care-delivery standards. The group is home to the National Long-Term Care Ombudsman Resources Center, and serves as a clearinghouse for current information on institutional-based long-term care. Consumers may request a list of publications available for sale.

Support Housing for the Elderly

Programs offered through the US Department of Housing and Urban Development (HUD) can help older people find affordable housing. For information, contact your local HUD office, listed in the blue pages of your local telephone directory.

Mental Health

American Association of Suicidology
4201 Connecticut Avenue, NW, Suite 408
Washington, DC 20008
phone: (202) 237-2280
fax: (202) 237-2282
web site: http://www.suicidology.org

The American Association of Suicidology (AAS) is a nonprofit organization dedicated to the understanding and prevention of suicide. The AAS promotes research, public awareness programs, education, and training for mental health professionals, suicide survivors, students, and volunteers. The association develops certification standards for suicide prevention and crisis centers and evaluates crisis workers for certification in crisis management. The organization serves as a national clearinghouse for information on suicide. AAS membership is open to mental health organizations, mental health professionals, students, volunteers, and anyone with an interest in suicide prevention or life-threatening behaviors. Contact the AAS for free information on suicide and suicide prevention and nationwide referrals to suicide prevention and crisis centers and support groups.

American Psychiatric Association
1400 K Street, NW
Washington, DC 20005
phone: (888) 357-7924
fax: (202) 682-6850
web site: http://www.psych.org

The American Psychiatric Association (APA) is a professional organization of physicians who specialize in psychiatry. The association offers information on mental health issues and referrals to state psychiatric societies, which can make referrals to local psychiatrists. The APA Web site offers online versions of two different types of APA pamphlets for consumers: *Let's Talk Facts About* and *APA Fact Sheets*. A number of topics are available online, including Alzheimer's disease, depression, coping with HIV and AIDS, substance abuse, teen suicide, and memories of sexual abuse. For a complete list of available pamphlets and for information on ordering hard-copy versions, access the APA Web site, or send your request to the association at the address above.

American Psychological Association
750 First Street, NE
Washington, DC 20002-4242
phone: (800) 374-2721 or (202) 336-5500
web site: http://www.apa.org

The American Psychological Association (APA) is the world's largest association of psychologists. APA works for the advancement of psychology as a science, as a profession, and as a means of promoting human welfare and provides free referrals to local practitioners nationwide. The APA publishes a variety of brochures and pamphlets on mental health topics of interest to consumers, including *Breast Cancer: How Your Mind Can Help Your Body; Controlling Anger—Before It Controls You;* and *Managing Traumatic Stress: Tips for Recovering from Disasters and Other Traumatic Events*. The APA also publishes a series of children's books on a wide variety of topics to help children deal with the issues they may confront—including adoption and foster care, depression, divorce, school problems, and self-esteem. Contact the APA for a referral or for more information about obtaining APA publications.

AMI Quebec

5253 Decarie Boulevard, Suite 150
Montreal, Quebec
H3W 3C3
phone: (514) 486-1448
fax: (514) 486-6157
web site: http://www.dsuper.net/~amique

AMI Quebec (Alliance for the Mentally Ill, Inc.) is a grassroots support and advocacy group that serves the families and friends of people who are mentally ill. AMI Quebec works to eliminate the shame and stigma associated with mental illness by raising public awareness. AMI Quebec offers a variety of self-help groups, seminars, education programs, and other resources, primarily for the English-speaking population. AMI Quebec also advocates legislation for protection and quality care for people with mental illness and promotes research on treatment, rehabilitation, and cure.

National Institute of Mental Health

Public Inquiries
6001 Executive Boulevard, Room 8184, MSC 9663
Bethesda, MD 20892-9663
phone: (301) 443-4513
fax: (301) 443-4279
web site: http://www.nimh.nih.gov

The National Institute of Mental Health (NIMH) is part of the National Institutes of Health, the principal biomedical and behavioral research agency of the US government. The National Institutes of Health is part of the US Department of Health and Human Services. The NIMH is dedicated to achieving better understanding, treatment, and prevention of mental illness through research. The institute offers a wide variety of brochures, information sheets, reports, press releases, fact sheets, and other educational materials that contain the latest information about symptoms, diagnosis, and treatment of various mental illnesses, including anxiety disorders, bipolar disorder, depression, learning disabilities, and obsessive-compulsive disorder. Consumers may access this and other useful information on the NIMH Web site or call or write the NIMH for additional information.

Rehabilitation

American Physical Therapy Association
Section on Geriatrics
1111 North Fairfax Street
Alexandria, VA 22314-1488
phone: (703) 684-APTA (2782)
fax: (703) 684-7343
web site: http://www.geriatricspt.org/consumer/ggeneral.html

The American Physical Therapy Association (APTA) is a professional organization dedicated to the advancement of physical therapy practice, research, and education. The APTA's section on geriatrics offers helpful information for older consumers, including an overview of physical therapy and its potential benefits, a state-by-state listing of physical therapists who have been certified as geriatric specialists by the APTA, and other resources, including tips on exercise, taking care of your back, and dealing with incontinence.

National Rehabilitation Information Center
1010 Wayne Avenue, Suite 800
Silver Springs, MD 20910
phone: (800) 346-2742 or (301) 562-2400 or
    (301) 495-5626 (TTY)
fax: (301) 562-2401
web site: http://www.naric.com/naric

The National Rehabilitation Information Center (NARIC) is funded by the National Institute on Disability and Rehabilitation Research of the US Department of Education. The NARIC provides information and referral services for anyone interested in mental and physical disability and rehabilitation. You may call, write, or visit the facility in person to request information and referrals at no cost. The NARIC's extensive collection of publications includes books, journal articles, pamphlets, audiovisual materials, and more. The NARIC can perform database searches for materials on specific topics and provide photocopies of those materials (within the limits of current US copyright law). Most NARIC publications (including materials obtained through database searches) are also available in large-print, audiocassette, and braille format; all NARIC documents are available on PC-compatible diskettes.

Self-help and Support

American Self-Help Clearinghouse
100 Hanover Avenue, Suite 202
Cedar Knolls, NJ 07927-2020
phone: (973) 326-6789
fax: (973) 326-9467
web site: http://www.selfhelpgroups.org

The American Self-Help Clearinghouse offers access to information on more than 800 national and international self-help and support groups through its searchable online database, Self-Help Sourcebook Online. The clearinghouse also publishes a hardcopy version, *Self-Help Sourcebook*, which is available for purchase by mail.

Catholic Golden Age
430 Penn Avenue
Scranton, PA 18503
phone: (800) 836-5699 or (570) 586-1091

Catholic Golden Age is a charitable organization that helps older people meet their physical, intellectual, social, economic, and spiritual needs. The organization offers group insurance plans and discounts on eyeglasses, prescriptions, and travel to its members. Programs conducted by local chapters include health promotion and disease prevention. Catholic Golden Age also publishes a bimonthly newsletter.

Children of Aging Parents
1609 Woodbourne Road, Suite 302-A
Levittown, PA 19057
phone: (800) 227-7294 or (215) 945-6900
fax: (215) 945-8720
web site: http://www.careguide.net

Children of Aging Parents (CAPS) is a nonprofit membership

organization for people who are caring for aging relatives. CAPS conducts workshops for community groups to promote understanding of the special needs of older people and offers training programs for nurses and social workers in hospitals, nursing facilities, and rehabilitation centers. The organization is a clearinghouse for information on resources for older people; call its information and referral service to learn about support groups and other resources available in your community. CAPS publishes a newsletter, *Capsule*, for members, and produces brochures and fact sheets for caregivers.

Choice in Dying

National Office
1035 30th Street, NW
Washington, DC 20007
phone: (800) 989-WILL (9455) or (202) 338-9790
fax: (202) 338-0242
web site: http://www.choices.org

Choice in Dying is a nonprofit organization that assists patients and their families with end-of-life medical care decision-making. The organization provides state-specific living will and durable power of attorney forms for a nominal fee; counsels patients and their families; educates and advises through its publications and training and outreach programs; and supports patients' rights legislation at both state and federal levels.

Disabled American Veterans

National Service and Legislative Headquarters
807 Maine Avenue, SW
Washington, DC 20024
phone: (202) 554-3501
web site: http://www.dav.org

Disabled American Veterans (DAV) is a private, nonprofit organization that helps veterans who have service-related disabilities and their families. Services provided include counseling, employment programs, help in obtaining free healthcare, and assistance with filing claims for veterans' benefits such as disability compensation and pensions. The Older Veterans Assistance Program offers additional assistance to older veterans and their families. A list of free publications is available from state DAV service offices; check your local phone book or call the number listed above to locate the DAV office that serves your state.

Friends' Health Connection
P.O. Box 114
New Brunswick, NJ 08903
phone: (800) 483-7436
fax: (732) 249-9897
web site: http://www.48friend.org

For a modest fee, Friends' Health Connection, a nonprofit organization, matches people who have health problems with other people who have similar health problems to enable them to provide friendship and support to each other. Friends' Health Connection's Family Network provides a similar service for caregivers, family members, and friends of people who have health problems. Such relationships can be established via mail, telephone, or e-mail.

National Easter Seal Society
230 West Monroe Street, Suite 1800
Chicago, IL 60606
phone: (800) 221-6827 or (312) 726-6200 or (312) 726-4258 (TDD)
fax: (312) 726-1494
web site: http://www.easter-seals.org

The National Easter Seal Society (Easter Seals) is a nationwide, community-based organization that serves children and adults with disabilities and their families. Easter Seals provides services such as preschool, daycare, after-school care, camp, respite care, job training, job placement, mentoring, medical screening, rehabilitation, and support.

Self Help for Hard of Hearing People, Inc.
7910 Woodmont Avenue, Suite 1200
Bethesda, MD 20814
phone: (301) 657-2248 or (301) 657-2249 (TTY)
fax: (301) 913-9413
web site: http://www.shhh.org

Self Help for Hard of Hearing People, Inc. (SHHH) is an organization that works to improve the quality of life for people with impaired hearing through education, advocacy, and self-help. SHHH publishes a quarterly newsletter, *SHHH News*, and a bimonthly magazine, *Hearing Loss: The Journal of Self Help for Hard of Hearing People*. The organization provides guidance and support for people of all ages with hearing loss and for parents of children with hearing loss. SHHH also offers consumers and professionals a wide variety of publications on topics related to hearing loss, including prevention, detection, coping, hearing aids, and effective communication. Local chapters of SHHH offer support and encouragement to people with hearing loss and provide information about and referrals to community resources.

Well Spouse Foundation
30 East 40th Street PH
New York, NY 10016
phone: (800) 838-0879 or (212) 685-8815
fax: (212) 685-8676
web site: http://www.wellspouse.org

Well Spouse Foundation is a nonprofit self-help organization that offers support for people who are caring for a chronically ill or disabled spouse. The organization helps to educate healthcare professionals, politicians, and the general public about long-term care and the needs of caregivers. Well Spouse Foundation publishes a bimonthly newsletter and sponsors an annual weekend conference for its members. The organization also provides personal outreach to its members through calls, letters, and ongoing support for members whose spouses have died.

Senior Advocacy

American Association of Retired Persons
601 E Street, NW
Washington, DC 20049
phone: (800) 424-3410
web site: http://www.aarp.org

The American Association of Retired Persons (AARP) is a membership group that serves the needs of people age 50 and over with information, education, advocacy, and community services. There are local AARP chapters throughout the United States, and membership is open to people who have not yet retired. AARP publishes *Modern Maturity* magazine and the monthly *AARP Bulletin* and offers information on a wide variety of topics of interest to older people, including caregiving, long-term care, housing, and financial planning. An AARP membership card entitles enrollees to many different discounts on travel expenses and other purchases.

Asociacion Nacional Pro Personas Mayores
(National Association for Hispanic Elderly)
1452 West Temple Street, Suite 100
Los Angeles, CA 90026
phone: (213) 202-5900
fax: (213) 202-5905

Asociacion Nacional Pro Personas Mayores (ANPPM) is an advocacy group that promotes recognition of the needs of older Hispanic people and ensures that they have access to social service programs. The ANPPM provides training and technical assistance to community groups and professionals in the field of gerontology (the study of aging). The group conducts market studies and research on aging in the Hispanic community through its National Hispanic Research Center, and publishes and distributes bilingual (Spanish/English) information on older Hispanic people through its Hispanic Media Center. The Senior Community Service Employment Program, which is funded by the US Department of Labor and administered by the ANPPM, employs low-income people 55 years of age and older in eight states and Puerto Rico. The ANPPM also provides information, referrals, and direct social services, and publishes articles, brochures, and audiovisual materials on Social Security, Medicare, and health-related topics.

B'nai B'rith
1640 Rhode Island Avenue, NW
Washington, DC 20036-3278
phone: (202) 857-6589
fax: (202) 857-1099
The Center for Senior Housing and Services: (202) 857-6581
Travel/Volunteer Programs: (800) 500-6533

web site: http://www.bnaibrith.org

B'nai B'rith, the oldest and largest Jewish service organization in the world, is dedicated to community service, Jewish education, and public advocacy. The B'nai B'rith Center for Senior Housing and Services sponsors and maintains nonsectarian federally subsidized housing for senior citizens; conducts continuing education, recreation, and other activities and events; and advocates on behalf of issues of importance to older people in cooperation with the B'nai B'rith Center for Public Policy. B'nai B'rith also sponsors travel and travel-volunteer programs for senior citizens and their families.

Catholic Charities USA
1731 King Street, Suite 200
Alexandria, VA 22314
phone: (703) 549-1390
fax: (703) 549-1656
web site: http://www.catholiccharitiesusa.org

Catholic Charities USA is a nationwide social service organization that provides assistance to people of all ages and backgrounds who are in need. The organization offers a wide range of services for older people, such as counseling, homemaker services, foster family programs, group homes and institutional care, public access programs, caregiver services, and emergency assistance and shelter. Catholic Charities USA also works to advance the rights of older people with regard to employment, housing, and Social Security benefits.

Gray Panthers
733 15th Street, NW, Suite 437
Washington, DC 20005
phone: (800) 280-5362 or (202) 737-6637
fax: (202) 737-1160

Gray Panthers is an advocacy group that works toward social change for the benefit of older people and others in regard to factors such as healthcare, housing, environment, education, and attitudes about aging. Local chapters sponsor public education seminars and organize groups of younger and older people to work together on important social issues. Gray Panthers offers information and referral services for resources for older people. The group also gathers and distributes information on research in gerontology (the study of aging). Members receive *NETWORK Newsletter*, a bimonthly newsletter. Call or write to request a list of publications.

National Academy of Elder Law Attorneys, Inc.
1604 North Country Club Road
Tucson, AZ 85716
phone: (520) 881-4005
fax: (520) 325-7925
web site: http://www.naela.com

The National Academy of Elder Law Attorneys, Inc. is a nonprofit professional organization that provides information, education, assistance, and networking for lawyers and others who work with older people and their families. The academy can refer you to a lawyer in your area who specializes in handling legal matters that are of particular concern to older people.

National Asian Pacific Center on Aging
Melbourne Tower
1511 3rd Avenue, Suite 914
Seattle, WA 98101
phone: (206) 624-1221
fax: (206) 642-1023
web site: http://www.napca.org

The National Asian Pacific Center on Aging (NAPCA) is a private, nationwide organization dedicated to improving healthcare and social services for older people who are members of the Asian Pacific community in the United States. The center provides assistance to community groups, maintains a national network of service agencies, conducts workshops and training programs for healthcare and social service professionals, and provides information and referral for family and community support groups. The center also employs older people through its nationwide Seniors' Community Service Employment Program. The organization's available publications include *Asian Pacific Affairs* (published bimonthly) and *The Registry of Services for Asian Pacific Elders*. The NAPCA Web site includes Chinese translations of official Medicare documents.

National Association of Professional Geriatric Care Managers
1604 North Country Club Road
Tucson, AZ 85716-3102
phone: (520) 881-8008
fax: (520) 325-7925

The National Association of Professional Geriatric Care Managers is a professional organization dedicated to promoting high-quality, cost-effective healthcare and human services for older people and their families. The association publishes a nationwide referral directory of professional geriatric care managers, which is available for sale.

National Council on the Aging, Inc.
409 3rd Street, SW
Washington, DC 20024
phone: (202) 479-1200
fax: (202) 479-0735
web site: http://www.ncoa.org

The National Council on the Aging (NCOA) is a private, non-profit organization that serves as a resource for information on all aspects of aging, including technical assistance, training, advocacy, and leadership for service providers and consumers. The NCOA publishes a wide range of literature on topics of interest to older people, their families, and healthcare professionals. The organization is especially knowledgeable about senior centers, adult day care, long-term care, senior housing, and issues that affect older people who live in rural areas. The National Institute on Adult Daycare is part of the NCOA.

National Senior Citizens Law Center
(Washington, DC office)
1101 14th Street, NW, Suite 400
Washington, DC 20005

phone: (202) 289-6976
fax: (202) 289-7224

(Los Angeles office)
3435 Wilshire Boulevard, Suite 2860
Los Angeles, CA 90010-1938
phone: (213) 639-0930
fax: (213) 639-0934
web site: http://www.nsclc.org

The National Senior Citizens Law Center (NSCLC) is a public-interest law firm established to meet the legal needs (including issues dealing with Social Security, Medicare, Medicaid, age discrimination, pension rights, home healthcare, and nursing facilities) of low-income older people. The NSCLC does not usually handle individual clients but provides information, referrals, and consulting services and technical assistance to legal aid offices and attorneys in private practice who serve older, low-income clients. A variety of helpful manuals and reference documents for consumers are available from the NSCLC for a nominal charge. To consult with an NSCLC attorney, write or fax a full description of your legal problem to the appropriate address above. You *must* include your full name, address, and telephone number in all correspondence with the NSCLC. Be sure, also, to include a description (including dates) of any contact you have had with an attorney about your problem.

National Women's Health Network
514 10th Street, NW, Suite 400
Washington, DC 20004
phone: (202) 347-1140 or (202) 628-7814
fax: (202) 347-1168

The National Women's Health Network is dedicated to ensuring that women have access to quality, affordable healthcare. The network also serves as a clearinghouse of information on women's health issues. Members receive a bimonthly newsletter that contains information about women's health topics and the network's lobbying efforts for women's health.

Miscellaneous

Alliance of Claims Assistance Professionals
731 Naperville Road
Wheaton, IL 60187-6407
phone: (630) 588-1260
fax: (630) 690-0377
web site: http://www.claims.org

The Alliance of Claims Assistance Professionals is a national, non-profit professional organization that can help you locate experienced professionals in your area who can assist you with processing health insurance claims.

Medic Alert
2323 Colorado Avenue
Turlock, CA 95382-2018
phone: (800) 432-5378
fax: (209) 669-2450
web site: http://www.medicalert.org

Medic Alert is a nonprofit membership organization that provides identification and medical information in emergencies. Each member wears an identification bracelet or pendant bearing an emblem that indicates the wearer has a hidden medical condition or needs special medical treatment in emergency situations. He or she also carries a wallet card that contains up-to-date personal medical information. The emblem alerts emergency workers and others to vital medical facts about the person and instructs them to contact a 24-hour Emergency Response Center where trained personnel provide lifesaving information. Medic Alert bracelets and pendants are particularly helpful for people who have allergies, chronic conditions such as diabetes, epilepsy, Parkinson's disease, or Alzheimer's disease, or who take medications. Medic Alert charges a modest yearly fee for membership.

**National Center for Chronic Disease Prevention
  and Health Promotion**
Tobacco Information and Prevention Source
Publications Catalog, Mail Stop K-50
4770 Buford Highway, NE
Atlanta, GA 30341-3717
phone: (800) 232-1311 or (770) 488-5705
fax: (888) 232-3299 (automated fax information service)
web site: http://www.cdc.gov/tobacco

The National Center for Chronic Disease Prevention and Health Promotion offers a wide variety of materials and information for people with hypertension. The Tobacco Information and Prevention Source (TIPS) provides publications on smoking and health as well as information about quitting smoking.

Index